THE ENEGY BOOST

Increase your Energy levels in 7 days

Federica Lippi

INDEX

INTRODUCTION

it is one of the ironies of modern life at a time when medical advances allow us to overcome so many of the problems that were once thought of as incurable and the technology is available to make all our lives so much easier, life in reality has never been more difficult.

This is reflected in so many different ways, some minor but many far less so meaning that for millions of people all over the world, just getting through the day feels like it's a major achievement.

There are of course many reasons why this can happen as life does not always treat us the way we would like it to, but one common complaint nowadays is that people often feel that they have a lack of energy, not enough "get up and go" to successfully navigate through whatever their daily routine throws in their direction. And although health, fitness and wellness is now a huge online business, it is for example generally agreed that "weight loss" information is the second most searched for subject on the net, there is surprisingly little information about energy and more specifically about how you can increase your energy levels.

In fact, what you are going to read in this book could literally change your life because once you know how to increase the levels of energy available to you, then it becomes far easier to ensure that you never again find yourself in a place where you feel permanently tired and drained of energy no matter what you seem to do. There is one thing to appreciate before we start however.

The reason this book focuses on a 7 day program is that replacing energy that has apparently trickled away over the years is not something that is going to happen overnight because there are no quick fixes. In fact, the very thing that most people would probably think as being capable of supplying a quick "energy bust" will often leave you feel more tired than ever as you will discover later. At the same time, this does not mean that it is going to take a full 7 days to feel any benefits. As soon as you start making appropriate changes that you are going to read of here, you are likely to begin to feel increasingly energetic pretty quickly but of course, every person is different.

Nevertheless, if a lack of energy is a big problem, what you are just about to read could be life changing.

What's the problem ?

When researching this book, one thing that became clear very quickly was that there are many different reasons why an individual might feel tired or fatigued.

However, one common feature of the majority people who are asking questions about why they feel almost permanently tired on the web (and using other resources like magazines and newspaper) is the fact most of these people are trying to live a healthy life, exactly the kind of life that suggest that a lack of energy should not be a problem for them.

And yet, they are suffering, so it does not appear that living in a healthy way is good enough to stave off fatigue and tiredness on its own. It is therefore necessary to examine what other contributory factors there might be as it will no doubt help to combat fatigue. If you can establish why you feel so tired and listless in the first place.

Some of the factors that serve to reduce the energy available to power your body through the day or to limit your body's ability to use the available energy efficiently are as follows:

A lack of sleep: it should be fairly obvious that is you do not get enough sleep every night, you are inevitability going to feel fatigued and listless throughout the following day. In addition however, there is also an unfortunate cumulative effect if you are not getting enough sleep. In this case, it is fairly inevitable that the fatigue you feel every day will gradually increase as the energy deficit takes an ever-increasing toll on your capacity to perform at the top of your game.

Stress: stress is something that is almost unavoidable in the high paced modern world we live in but this does not mean that it is either acceptable or unavoidable. Stress can never be acceptable because it is a condition that is often at the root of a very wide range of medical problems (both physical and psychological). On top of this , it does not have to be something that you accept either as you will discover later in the book. Even so, it is the fact of 21st-century life that stress hits most of us at some time or other (for some people, it is every day) and it is therefore essential to understand that stress is going to make you feel far less energetic that you might otherwise be for several reasons. Firstly, if you have ever gone to bed immediately after a big arguments, you will already be aware that when your brain is still hot-wired after such a contretemps, it is impossible to go to sleep quickly. You are still stressed, your nerves are on edge and the adrenaline is still pumping, so the chances of getting to sleep in this mental state are fairly minimal. Secondly, being stressed makes your body less efficient whilst the nervous energy that we would normally associate with being tense and stressed is energy that is being leached from more positive usage. When you are uptight and stressed, your body is producing large amounts of hormones, a process which itself uses up a significant amount of energy that you would otherwise have available to help you through the day. This is why being stressed and uptight is likely to leave you feeling drained and shattered immediately afterwards as the energy high that has been driving your highly excited state quickly falls away.

Nutrient food deficit: The fact that our modern diet is responsible for an ever expanding range of health problems (or perhaps more accurately, deficiencies) might come as a surprise to some people. After all, they see an ever expanding range seemingly delicious, nutritious foods on the shelves in the local hypermarket, or store, a lot of which is increasingly affordable, so they quite naturally assume that our modern diet should provide all of the goodness and nutrients that we need. Unfortunately, however, nothing could be further from the truth for many different reasons.

Firstly, the fact that people want,(or maybe need) the price of the weekly food shopping to keep falling puts a great deal of pressure on commercial food manufacturers to increase efficiency and output levels.

Consequently, the quality of food products that you buy almost incessantly fall as a direct result of wanting to pay less for bananas and/or beefsteak than you were paying before. As an example, imagine that you are planning to purchase a commercially produced fruit pie. If you want that pie to contain only top quality, high nutritious fruit and other materials, then the price you will have to pay will reflect the quality of the content of the product. If however, you want to pay a rock bottom price, then quite obviously, the quality of the content will also be reflected in the price, meaning that the fruit included is nowhere near as nutritious or healthy as it could have been. Even with something as humble as a simple fruit pie, there is however a chain of production and at every stage of that chain, economics have to be made and shortcuts need to be taken as well.

For instance, the farmer who grew that fruit is being pushed by the pie manufacturer to produce increasingly cheap fruit for his pies, this means that the farmer has to produce more than before to keep his business afloat. Consequently, he (or she) turns to chemical fertilizers and insecticides to make sure that the business is capable of producing a maximum amount of produce from every square meter of land that is being farmed. However you want to cut it, there are no safe chemicals fertilizers or insecticides. Not only these chemicals pollute the environment whilst altering pH balance of the soil so that it becomes increasingly infertile and toxic, they destroy the healthy microorganism in the soil which is basically where the goodness in the food you eat should come from.

Furthermore, chemicals take carrying amounts of time to break down, with some becoming increasingly toxic as they do so. These poisons can stay in the soil (which is going to be growing even more fruit or other crops next year) and in the water supply (the same water you may be drinking right now) for many years to come. There are other problems too. Whilst every amateur gardener understand that insects can be a nuisance when you're trying to grow any kind of plant, it is still a fact that only about 6% of species of insects carry any kind of threat. Unfortunately, chemical insecticides are entirely indiscriminate, meaning that they kill both the good and bad insects, which is becoming an increasing concern for scientists who are seeing the balance of nature being indelibly shifted. These chemicals can even creep into the meat element of your diet as cows and sheep graze on pasture under which the soil has been damaged by many years of chemical ministration. Other creatures such as pigs and chicken are given feed that is likely to be tainted in the same way.

Improperly prepared food : Another factor that you need to take into account when looking at the genuine value of your diet is the fact that whether you are eating at home or in a restaurant, the changes are that food preparation methods you (or the chef) use are designed more for convenience that they are for retaining the nutrients that exist in the food being prepared.

For instance, whenever you boil vegetables, you remove a significantly percentage of the nutrients from them which are then tipped away with the water after you have finished cooking. Instead of boiling vegetables, it therefore makes a great deal more sense in nutritional terms to steam them so that they retain the goodness as steam leaches for less of the available nutrients than does surrounding them with boiling water.

Frying food is not a particularly good option either as doing so adds extra fat to your food which is not really something you want to do. A quick sauté in a healthy unsalted oil such as virgin version extracted from olives may not be too bad but frying food for several minutes in a less healthy oil all but guaranteed that you food absorbs a percentage of that oil. Which is very bad for your all-round health.

Another thing to appreciate when considering the nutrients in your food is that some nutrients (or a lack of them) have been directly linked to fatigue and listlessness. For example, the main types of anemia are caused by shortages of iron, vitamin B12 and folic acid, all of which are needed to produce red blood cells.

Anemia is a condition that is most commonly seen in pregnant women or those who suffer an unusually heavy monthly cycle, but if you are anemic for any reason and these nutrients are missing from your food, it could be a major cause of a constant feeling of being tired.

Drugs by the "back door": There is another extremely important consideration when it comes to meat products, something that very few people are actively aware of. In many develop Western countries, it is increasingly common for commercial farmers to feed drugs to their livestock to make sure that the creatures they are breeding for meat gain the maximum amount of weight possible and that they stay disease-free-

The additional weight being ladled on to these poor animals is almost completely water, meaning that an increasingly large percentage of your meat shopping bill is buying you nothing more than plain water.

The fact is, farm animals are increasingly pumped full of (or fed) drugs such as antibiotics, hormones and steroids in an effort to keep them disease-free, maximize their weight and so on. As a result, if you eat meat products without really knowing what is in them, the chances are that you are consuming an unknown amount of unidentified antibiotics and other drugs without even knowing it.

Nowadays, it is a recognized fact that the citizens of most Western countries are far too over-reliant on antibiotic drugs, primarily because for several decades, the first choice of most doctors when confronted with a sick patient has been to prescribe this particular form of drug. Although doctors all over the world are happy to prescribe antibiotics for a wide range of conditions (although there is some evidence that this may be becoming less common) including such thing as influenza, whereas influenza is caused by a virus, meaning that antibiotics will make no difference whatsoever.

However, because antibiotics have been so rashly overused for such an extended period of time and because bacteria mutate on a regular basis, there are now many strains of bacteria that are entirely resistant to most or all antibiotic drugs.

The bottom line here is, irrespective of how careful you are about taking antibiotic drugs unless it is absolutely necessary, you could inadvertently be ingesting antibiotics and other potentially harmful drugs every time you sit down to the dinner table.

The problem you must therefore understand is that whilst you might be trying to eat a healthy diet that is theoretically capable of providing all of the energy you need, it does not follow that because all of the food on the table appears to be nutritious that it really is. Consequently, it is a fact that many people who suffer a lack of energy every day could be falling foul of the tricks of the food production industry. And of course, if this is the case, the chemicals and drugs that you are taking on board could be exacerbating the problems that leave you feeling listless and fatigued because of problems like stress and a lack of sleep.

Western medicine : As highlighted in the previous section, it is now widely accepted that for many decades, people have been far too willing to take a huge cocktail of prescription drugs that were given to them by their doctor or medical care professional, usually on the basis that "doctors always know best". And whilst there is no doubt that in the majority of cases, the drugs prescribed were entirely appropriate to the condition being treated, this has not always been the case. Hence, you may have built up an internal residue of chemicals over the years that are at least partially responsible for your general feeling of ennui.

Furthermore, because Western medicine focuses on dealing with the symptoms of illness and disease rather than on getting to the root cause of the problem before dealing with it at that level, many conditions that people suffer from never leave them or allow them to return to or retain 100% good health. This lack of conditioning can be seen in many different ways, with a constant feeling of being tired one of the most common.

Your environment: The environment that surrounds you every day is likely to have a very significant effect on your general state of health and wellness as well for a wide variety of reasons.

For example, whilst air-pollution is perhaps not as endemic as it was 50 years ago, it is still a major problem if you happen to live in a large town or majority city. If you're surrounded by motor vehicles every day, the vast majority are still pumping out poisonous carbon monoxide fumes, which naturally means that you are breathing these potentially noxious substances every day.

Furthermore, whilst there are millions of people all over the world who might be termed "sun worshippers", having the sun beating down on the top of your head every day is not always a good time. There are many side-effects and potential illness associated with too much sunshine (e.g. skin cancer).

On the other hand, everyone needs sunshine on their skin from time to time because without it, you have no chance of creating vitamin D (which is produced by the effects of the sun on your skin) which is in turn responsible for regulating the ability of your body to absorb an use calcium efficiently. If your body in not using minerals and trace elements properly, this is extremely likely to contribute to your general feeling of tiredness.

There are also people who suffer a recognized form of depression known as Seasonal Affective Disorder that strikes people in the depths of winter when sunlight is at a premium. One of the most commonly reported effects of this condition is a lack of energy and a general disinterest in life, something that passes for 99% of sufferers once the spring arrives and the sun appears over the horizon once again.

Where you live, what season it is and everything that surrounds you can therefore have a significant role to play in dictating how much energy you have available.

Your physical condition: I would suggest that it should be pretty obvious to most people that if you are badly out of shape, you are inevitably going to feel as if you lack energy and the "get up and go" to do something about remedying the situation. However, the fact that nearly 40% of the adult population is obese (a percentage which is exploding) tends to suggest that my assumption may not be completely accurate! It is nevertheless a fact that if you are overweight and do not do any exercise, then without making significant lifestyle changes, your lack of energy is a problem that is never likely to be remedied. Whilst carrying too much weight does not guarantee that you will lack energy per se (some of the most successful bodybuilders carry more weight than they should, but it is "good" muscle weight), for the majority who have a weight problem, a lack of energy is pretty much a given byproduct of their condition.

101 combinations: The reason that I have put forward for why you might suffer from a lack of energy so far could suggest that there is going to be one reason or another that you can really identify that is entirely responsible for your condition. However, the fact is that in the majority of cases, it will be causing the way you feel and not all of these reasons might be apparent or included in this list, mainly because every person who feels tired does so for different reasons (and more often than not because of a combination of them). For instance, if you are stressed, then it is likely that you're not sleeping very well and that you are probably not concentrating on eating a healthy diet quite as much as you should be. Hence, there are three factors that between them are causing you to feel the way you do, although it is probable that in this situation, one problem is leading to the others.

Nevertheless, if you understand that a problem like a lack of energy is likely to be caused by a combination of factors, the way that you deal with the situation should become that much clearer.

BEGIN AT THE BEGINNING

Although the previous chapter is designed to help you identify some of the factors that might have a part to play in dictating how drained you feel every day, it is important to understand that these are only intended to be a general guideline to get you started and definitely not a detailed medical opinion. However, if you do suffer from a lack of energy that blights your life every day, perhaps the most important thing to do is find out exactly why you feel the way you do. And there is no sense in guessing here because you have to establish whether there is any specific reason why you feel the way you do before you can concentrate on increasing your energy levels in a more general, all round way.

In other words, the first thing that you should do if you feel that you lack energy or that each day is becoming increasingly difficult to get through is make an appointment with your doctor or other medical care professional to seek their advice to establish whether there is a genuine underlying medical condition causing you problems.

If you feel okay but just would like to become more energetic, then it's probably not necessary to seek the doctor's advice but if on the other hand you feel constantly tired, there may be a specific medical reason for the condition that needs to be identified before deciding upon the most effective form of remedy. For instance, it was highlighted earlier that the main causes of anemia include a lack of iron, folic acid and vitamin B12. If you therefore have an anemia problem that is making you feel constantly tired, remedying the situation may involve nothing more complex than introducing more foods that are rich in these nutrients to your diet or using supplements to make sure that you have sufficient iron and vitamins to overcome the problem. If you genuinely feel that you consistently lack energy, having a word with your doctor seems to make a good deal of sense. At least in this way, you will either isolate the underlying problem so that it can be dealt with, or put your mind at rest that there is no such problem in the first place.

IT'S ABOUT YOUR LIFESTYLE
The seven-day program

Assuming that there is no underlying medical condition causing your lack of energy, you have arrived at the beginning of your seven-day program to increase your energy levels. This is the point from where you have to identify why you think you feel as if you lack energy because if you don0t do this, you cannot begin to make the necessary lifestyle changes that will see you rectifying the problem.

For instance, if you are a person who is always stressed, you probably have a major cause of your lack of energy pinned down already. A similar situation is likely to apply if you can see yourself in any of the "pen pictures" in the previous chapter, because you are badly out of shape, or overweight, you cannot realistically expect to be super energetic.

You therefore need to start thinking about how you go about remedying the situation that is causing you to suffer a lack of energy before going any further. This is important because whilst this book is focused on increasing your energy levels over a relatively short period of time, if you have to make large-scale lifestyle changes, it is likely to take a little more time before you feel the biggest benefits of making these changes. For example, despite adverts for commercial diet products that claim you can drop 10lbs or one clothes size per week, this is not going to happen for most people and even for those who do achieve success, the weight loss is almost entirely because they shed water. Moreover, weight lost in this way never stays away for the long term, so you need to think about this particular aspect of your program to increase energy levels in more depth.

In short, if you have obvious factors that are going to limit the likelihood of you feeling full of beans, energetic and vital every day, you must include specific measures to combat these limiting factors in your own seven-day energy increase program. If this is losing weight or reducing the amount of stress that you consciously feel, then you may want to focus on some aspects of what you are going to read in this book more than on others. However, whatever the reason is that you are currently lacking in energy, you will find a solution to your problem in the following chapters which will deal with your lack if energy both on a physical and psychological manner.

THE PHYSICAL SIDE IN GETTING MORE ENERGY

It is an oft bandied cliché that is nevertheless true that you are what you eat. In short, the physical "you" that you see staring back at you in the mirror in the morning is the sum total of every morsel of food and every liquid ounce of fluid you have ever consumed, which, taken to its logical conclusion, should tell you one thing.

If you don't have the energy that you think you should have, then the food and drinks that you have consumed thus far has not been capable of providing that energy for one reason or another.

What you therefore need to do is start making lifestyle changes that will turn the picture around so that in the future, the "you" that stares back in the mirror is made up of a very different "mix" to what you are made of now.

There are two ways that you should approach this problem, doing so in a macro-manner and also by managing your dietary intake on a micro. Level as well. Exactly what this means will become clearer as you continue reading, but your starting point is to view your daily food and drink consumption on a macro-basis by considering your diet as a whole.

MACRO-MANAGING YOUR DIET

If you are what you eat and you don't have enough energy, then your diet and lifestyle is either not providing the energy or not enabling you to release it as efficiently as you should, you therefore need to start making changes but before doing so, there is another vital factor to appreciate. The evolution of mankind is a relatively slow thing, which means that to all intents and purposes, our bodies and more importantly our metabolisms are still pretty much the way they were 1000 years ago. Sure, there have been some changes as we have (for example9 gradually become taller, but the fact is that our internal "workings" have not changed a great deal. However, our daily diet has changed by a massive amount, perhaps far more than you might ever have imagined, for example, whereas before the turn of the 20th century 8in 1890) the average western citizen consumed 5lbs of sugar a year, the figure is now 135lbs per annum, and that is up from 26lbs a little over 20 years ago ! Furthermore, as the diet of most citizens of developed nations has become increasingly focused on processed and convenience foods, our consumption of processed white flour, meat products of no determinable origin and the like have also skyrocketed. The results of these dietary changes have unfortunately been overwhelmingly negative in a huge number of different ways, most of which do us no favors. And the starting point for all these negative effects is the fact that the human digestive system has not adapted quickly enough to accept these changes and still be as efficient as it should be. What this means is that for most of us, our digestion is struggling to process the food that we feed into our system every day and whilst our digestive tract does a remarkably good job everything considered, it is unfortunately fighting a battle that can never win.

As a result of these changes, your gut or colon has gradually built up a store of toxins and noxious substances over the years that your digestive system does not have the ability to push through, most of these substances come from your diet, with others contributed by the environment (from the air you breathe), medical drugs and so on.

As these materials congregate in your colon, it naturally becomes less effective which in turn means that the buildup rate of toxic substances accelerates. It's a classic vicious circle because the more accumulated rubbish there is, the less efficient your system becomes so even more is acquired. Perhaps not surprisingly, all of the toxic material buildup inevitably slows you down and reduces your energy levels.

For instance, many millions of people suffer from constipation and/or diarrhea which are both classic signs that your colon is not in tiptop condition. Although to some people these symptoms are indicative of a recognized medical condition (e.g. Irritable Bowel Syndrome) for most it is highlighting the fact that you are not feeding your digestive system the foods and nutrients it needs. And whilst constipation and/or diarrhea might be unpleasant but no more, you should understand that they could indicate that you are more susceptible to far more serious medical problems such as colon cancer, which is one of the biggest killers in the Western world.

In short, your digestive system, colon and bowel are clogged up with toxic materials that are draining your energy in more ways than one.

For instance, you could be eating the most nutritious foods in the world but if your digestive system does not have the capability of processing them to extract all the nutrients, you are naturally enough not getting all of the benefits. There is therefore an immediate loss of energy and health here. This is further exacerbated by the fact that because your digestive system is packed with toxic materials, your body expends a significant amount of energy keeping the worst effects of these toxins in check. This is energy that your body is "stealing" from you in an effort to keep you healthy but is is nevertheless energy that you do not have access to. To put this into some kind of perspective, a healthy colon should weigh around 4lbs whereas some autopsy reports carried out on individuals who clearly lived a less than healthy life reported a 40lb colon! Not only would this have added a significant extra complication to any weight problems these individuals suffered, it is clear that their digestive system would have been all but incapable of doing its job.

When it comes to macro-managing your diet, there are therefore several considerations to take into account. The first thing that you must do if you want to increase your energy levels is to reduce the level of toxins /and other nasties like parasites) that are currently putting a significant drain on your energy resources. To do this, you might choose a commercially produced colon cleansing product, but this is not necessary, nor does it make a great deal of sense either when compared to natural dietary changes that will so the same thing.

The beauty of adopting a natural approach to getting rid of accumulated junk from your colon and bowels is that by doing so, you make changes that will help minimize the future buildup of these toxic materials as well. Getting rid of this accumulated toxic mélange in a natural manner and making sure that it doesn't return is one of the easiest and most effective ways of improving your energy levels, now, I am not going to pretend that you can remove this toxic mix from your body immediately, because it has taken years to accumulate so it is going to take a little time to shift it.

Even so , the changes take weeks rather than years and you will start to feel the benefits within days because optimum nutrition allows your system to rejuvenate itself extremely quickly and to extract the maximum amount of energy and vitality from the foods you consume. Let us therefore start to look exactly at what you should and what you should not be consuming if you want to increase your energy levels as quickly as possible.

THE DIETARY DON'TS

As suggested, the average citizen of most Wester countries consume a massive amount of processed sugar, which is just about the worst thing you can do for many different reasons. Some of these reasons are directly related to decreased energy levels, whereas others are more related to medical or physical problems that excessive sugar might cause which can also lead to low energy.

Most people probably understand that sucrose or processed white sugar is essentially pure energy, so they might therefore imagine that if you feel that your energy levels are low, eating sugar rich foods like candies, cookies, cakes and other sugary intakes believe that it's the perfect answer.

Unfortunately, this is the exact opposite of the truth because whilst a sugar rich food (or soft drink which is how most people consume the majority of their daily sugar intake) will give you an immediate "sugar high", it will also increase insulin levels which will bring you down again just as quickly. Sadly, many people find that after coming down from the sugar rush, they are even less energized and more tired that they were before, explaining exactly why consuming processed sugar is a transitory and relatively ineffective energy booster.

The potential problems caused by overconsumption of processed sugar do not however stop here. For example, most people are aware that vitamin C is an essential nutrient for continued good health but they may not be aware that one of the purposes it serves is to reduce the chances of cancer cells developing.

Unfortunately however, to do this, vitamin C must gain access to the white blood cells that combat cancer, and in this respect, they are in competition with sugar cells. Consequently, the more sugar you take on board, the less efficient vitamin C is able to be at preventing cancerous cells developing.

There is also evidence that too much sugar damages your immune system's ability to control your body efficiently and is believed that 80% of you immune system is focused on you digestion (where all the toxic rubbish is remember?), it should be clear that processed sugar is not a healthy source of energy by any stretch of the imagination. In a similar way, all other processed foods tend to have had most of the nutrients stripped from them. Sadly, the levels of more harmful substances like saturated fats (in burgers for example) have usually not been reduced whereas additional sugar has been introduced to enhance the flavor.

Once again, eating processed foods is not going to help to increase your energy levels, instead helping to pile up more of the toxic mountain lodged in your digestive tract that slows you down and steals your energy.

The bottom line here is, if you eat a diet that is rich in processed foods, sugar, saturated fats and the like, you are only encouraging the development of the noxious energy drain lodged in your digestive tract.

Do this and you cannot realistically hope to increase your energy levels, so don't do it. There is also the question of piling on the extra pounds to be considered as well. Because most overweight people (apart from those with a clinical reason for their condition know that it is a processed food diet that is most likely to make it even more difficult to get into their clothes.

WHAT SHOULD YOU DO ?

Okay, now we have looked at the "don't" side of a diet that will help you to increase your energy levels, let us consider what you should be eating, now !
The first thing that you must do is drink lots of fresh water. The minimum recommended water intake for everyone is at least eight glasses a day but as long as you don't go crazy, drinking more than this is a good idea, particularly during the first week when you're trying to get the energy boost ball rolling. Note that this is specifically water that you should be drinking (preferably alkaline water) and no other caffeine rich drinks like tea or coffee. Although some people find that caffeine gives them a boost, it is always a temporary one that needs replenishing on a regular basis, hence the idea of having a "coffee" habit. In a similar way to sugar rush, coming down from a caffeine high can also reduce your energy levels still further, so try to drink water as opposed to anything else.
However, one alternative beverage that you might include, especially in the early days when you are trying to detoxify your system is green tea, as it is believed that the polyphenols in the green tea help detoxify your body as well as playing a hand in preventing disease such as liver complaints and diabetes. There is plenty of

evidence that green tea is good for you in many ways, so including three or four cups of green tea in your new dietary regime every day would help to clear out your system, thereby increasing your energy levels.

To get started with your clean out, buy a good stock of organic fruit and vegetables that can be eaten raw. The idea of this is that for the first two or three days, the only foods that you should consume are raw fruits and vegetables to get your system "kick started".

As these organic products are high in nutrients, vitamins and trace minerals that your system has been missing, you should find that within 48 to 72 hour period, you already start to feel the benefits of this lifestyle change. At the same time however, you should not overdo things by eating too much as the idea is to minimize the strain on your digestive system whilst feeding it all the natural nutrients that help to normalize the balance in your colon and bowels.

To help take this one on the stage further, you should also include probiotic supplements in your new diet for this first week as these are the "good bacteria" without which your digestive and immune system are immeasurably weakened. As a result of the buildup of toxic garbage in your gut, the balance between good and bad bacteria has significantly shifted in favor of the lateral harmful variety, you need to start redress the balance by feeding your system probiotic bacteria. Incidentally, there are plenty of sites on the net where you can buy probiotic supplements, as all you need to do is run a standard google search to find somewhere suitable, or go to your local health food shop as they will have them too. Next, you should add psyllium seeds or husks to your diet as well as flax seeds as the first of these helps to neutralize the toxic effects of the buildup of waste as well as loosen the buildup materials, whereas the flax seeds absorb moisture whilst expanding in your colon, thereby helping to remove noxious substances and toxins.

Another substance that is often recommended a s a part of a short term detoxification diet is bentonite in liquid, powder or tablet form. This is a type of edible clay that acts as a bulk laxative that forms a gel after absorbing water in your gut. As it does so, it also absorbs many of the toxic materials that you're trying to shift, thereby accelerating the cleansing process.

If you stick to you "raw veggie" fast for two days or three days whilst taking the supplements shown, you should find that you feel a noticeable difference after you have finished. And whilst there is no particular harm in continuing to use the probiotics, seeds and bentonite tablets for a short period of time to optimize the internal cleansing process, you should not do so over the longer term. If you were to do this, your system may come to depend upon these "artificial stimulants" for good health, which is not something that you want to encourage.

However, fast for two or three days using only raw organic foods whilst also following this colon cleansing process and you will feel far more energetic and vital than you have felt in a long time.

Where to next ?

After you have cleaned out your system and you are feeling better than you have felt in months (or perhaps even years), I would guess that you do not want to go back to the situation where even getting out of bed in the morning seemed like a major task.

If not, you cannot afford to go back to your old dietary habits either because as the result of your "clean out" should have made obvious, it was those dietary habits that made you feel listless, fatigue and drained at the end of every day. What you must therefore do is adopt a healthy balanced diet rather than going back to the "bad old days", perhaps by following the guidelines of the "food pyramid".

My Plate illustrates the five food groups that are the building blocks for a healthy diet using a familiar image -- a place setting for a meal. Before you eat, think about what goes on your plate or in your cup or bowl.

FRUITS

What foods are in the Fruit Group?

Any fruit or 100% fruit juice counts as part of the Fruit Group. Fruits may be fresh, canned, frozen, or dried, and may be whole, cut-up, or pureed.

How much fruit is needed daily?

The amount of fruit you need to eat depends on age, sex, and level of physical activity. Recommended daily amounts are shown in the chart below.

Daily Fruit Chart		
Daily Recommendation*		
Children	2-3 years old	1 cup
	4-8 years old	1 to 1 1/2 cups
Girls	9-13 years old	1 1/2 cups
	14-18 years old	1 1/2 cups
Boys	9-13 years old	1 1/2 cups
	14-18 years old	2 cups
Women	19-30 years old	2 cups
	31-50 years old	1 1/2 cups

Daily Fruit Chart		
Daily Recommendation*		
	51+ years old	1 1/2 cups
Men	19-30 years old	2 cups
	31-50 years old	2 cups
	51+ years old	2 cups

*These amounts are appropriate for individuals who get less than 30 minutes per day of moderate physical activity, beyond normal daily activities. Those who are more physically active may be able to consume more while staying within calorie needs.

What counts as a cup of fruit?

In general, 1 cup of fruit or 100% fruit juice, or ½ cup of dried fruit can be considered as 1 cup from the Fruit Group. This chart below shows specific amounts that count as 1 cup of fruit (in some cases equivalents for ½ cup are also shown) towards your daily recommended intake.

Amount that counts as 1 cup of fruit		Other amounts (count as 1/2 cup of fruit unless noted)
Apple	1/2 large (3.25"	1/2 cup sliced or

Amount that counts as 1 cup of fruit		Other amounts (count as 1/2 cup of fruit unless noted)
	diameter)	chopped, raw or cooked
	1 small (2.5" diameter)	
	1 cup sliced or chopped, raw or cooked	
Applesauce	1 cup	1 snack container (4oz)
Banana	1 cup sliced	1 small (less than 6" long)
	1 large (8" to 9" long)	
Cantaloupe	1 cup diced or melon balls	1 medium wedge (1/8 of a med. melon)
Grapes	1 cup whole or cut-up	16 seedless grapes
	32 seedless grapes	
Grapefruit	1 medium (4" diameter)	1/2 medium (4" diameter)
	1 cup sections	
Mixed fruit (fruit cocktail)	1 cup diced or sliced, raw or canned, drained	1 snack container (4 oz) drained = 3/8 cup

Amount that counts as 1 cup of fruit		Other amounts (count as 1/2 cup of fruit unless noted)
Orange	1 large (3-1/16" diameter) 1 cup sections	1 small (2-3/8" diameter)
Orange, mandarin	1 cup canned, drained	
Peach	1 large (2 3/4" diameter) 1 cup sliced or diced, raw, cooked, or canned, drained 2 halves, canned	1 small (2" diameter) 1 snack container (4 oz) drained = 3/8 cup
Pear	1 medium pear (2.5 per lb) 1 cup sliced or diced, raw cooked, or canned, drained	1 snack container (4 oz) drained = 3/8 cup
Pineapple	1 cup chunks, sliced or crushed, raw, cooked or canned, drained	1 snack container (4 oz) drained = 3/8 cup
Plum	1 cup sliced raw	1 large plum

Amount that counts as 1 cup of fruit		Other amounts (count as 1/2 cup of fruit unless noted)
	or cooked 3 medium or 2 large plums	
Strawberries	About 8 large berries 1 cup whole, halved, or sliced, fresh or frozen	1/2 cup whole, halved, or sliced
Watermelon	1 small (1" thick) 1 cup diced or balls	6 melon balls

Dried fruit (raisins, prunes, apricots, etc.)	1/2 cup dried fruit is equivalent to 1 cup fruit:
	  1/2 cup raisins
	  1/2 cup prunes
	  1/2 cup dried apricots
		1/4 cup dried fruit is equivalent to 1/2 cup fruit 1 small box raisins (1.5 oz)

100% fruit juice (orange, apple, grape, grapefruit, etc.)	1 cup	1/2 cup

Why is it important to eat fruit?

Eating fruit provides health benefits — people who eat more fruits and vegetables as part of an overall healthy diet are likely to have a reduced risk of some chronic diseases. Fruits provide nutrients vital for health and maintenance of your body.

•Most fruits are naturally low in fat, sodium, and calories. None have cholesterol.
•Fruits are sources of many essential nutrients that are under consumed, including potassium, dietary fiber, vitamin C, and folate (folic acid).
•Diets rich in potassium may help to maintain healthy blood pressure. Fruit sources of potassium include bananas, prunes and prune juice, dried peaches and apricots, cantaloupe, honeydew melon, and orange juice.
•Dietary fiber from fruits, as part of an overall healthy diet, helps reduce blood cholesterol levels and may lower risk of heart disease. Fiber is important for proper bowel function. It helps reduce constipation and diverticulosis. Fiber-containing foods such as fruits help provide a feeling of fullness with fewer calories. Whole or cut-up fruits are sources of dietary fiber; fruit juices contain little or no fiber.
•Vitamin C is important for growth and repair of all body tissues, helps heal cuts and wounds, and keeps teeth and gums healthy.

•Folate (folic acid) helps the body form red blood cells. Women of childbearing age who may become pregnant should consume adequate folate from foods, and in addition 400 mcg of synthetic folic acid from fortified foods or supplements. This reduces the risk of neural tube defects, spina bifida, and anencephaly during fetal development.

Health benefits

•Eating a diet rich in vegetables and fruits as part of an overall healthy diet may reduce risk for heart disease, including heart attack and stroke.
•Eating a diet rich in some vegetables and fruits as part of an overall healthy diet may protect against certain types of cancers.
•Diets rich in foods containing fiber, such as some vegetables and fruits, may reduce the risk of heart disease, obesity, and type 2 diabetes.
•Eating vegetables and fruits rich in potassium as part of an overall healthy diet may lower blood pressure, and may also reduce the risk of developing kidney stones and help to decrease bone loss.
•Eating foods such as fruits that are lower in calories per cup instead of some other higher-calorie food may be useful in helping to lower calorie intake.

Tips to help you eat fruits

In general:
•Keep a bowl of whole fruit on the table, counter, or in

the refrigerator.
•Refrigerate cut-up fruit to store for later.
•Buy fresh fruits in season when they may be less expensive and at their peak flavor.
•Buy fruits that are dried, frozen, and canned (in water or 100% juice) as well as fresh, so that you always have a supply on hand.
•Consider convenience when shopping. Try pre-cut packages of fruit (such as melon or pineapple chunks) for a healthy snack in seconds. Choose packaged fruits that do not have added sugars.

For the best nutritional value:
•Make most of your choices whole or cut-up fruit rather than juice, for the benefits dietary fiber provides.
•Select fruits with more potassium often, such as bananas, prunes and prune juice, dried peaches and apricots, and orange juice.
•When choosing canned fruits, select fruit canned in 100% fruit juice or water rather than syrup.
•Vary your fruit choices. Fruits differ in nutrient content.
At meals:
•At breakfast, top your cereal with bananas or peaches; add blueberries to pancakes; drink 100% orange or grapefruit juice. Or, mix fresh fruit with plain fat-free or low-fat yogurt.
•At lunch, pack a tangerine, banana, or grapes to eat, or choose fruits from a salad bar. Individual containers of fruits like peaches or applesauce are easy and convenient.
•At dinner, add crushed pineapple to coleslaw, or

include orange sections or grapes in a tossed salad.
•Make a Waldorf salad, with apples, celery, walnuts, and a low-calorie salad dressing.
•Try meat dishes that incorporate fruit, such as chicken with apricots or mangoes.
•Add fruit like pineapple or peaches to kabobs as part of a barbecue meal.
•For dessert, have baked apples, pears, or a fruit salad.

As snacks:
•Cut-up fruit makes a great snack. Either cut them yourself, or buy pre-cut packages of fruit pieces like pineapples or melons. Or, try whole fresh berries or grapes.
•Dried fruits also make a great snack. They are easy to carry and store well. Because they are dried, ¼ cup is equivalent to ½ cup of other fruits.
•Keep a package of dried fruit in your desk or bag. Some fruits that are available dried include apricots, apples, pineapple, bananas, cherries, figs, dates, cranberries, blueberries, prunes (dried plums), and raisins (dried grapes).
•As a snack, spread peanut butter on apple slices or top plain fat-free or low-fat yogurt with berries or slices of kiwi fruit.
•Frozen juice bars (100% juice) make healthy alternatives to high-fat snacks.

Make fruit more appealing:
•Many fruits taste great with a dip or dressing. Try fat-free or low-fat yogurt as a dip for fruits like strawberries

or melons.

•Make a fruit smoothie by blending fat-free or low-fat milk or yogurt with fresh or frozen fruit. Try bananas, peaches, strawberries, or other berries.

•Try unsweetened applesauce as a lower calorie substitute for some of the oil when baking cakes.

•Try different textures of fruits. For example, apples are crunchy, bananas are smooth and creamy, and oranges are juicy.

•For fresh fruit salads, mix apples, bananas, or pears with acidic fruits like oranges, pineapple, or lemon juice to keep them from turning brown.

Fruit tips for children:

•Set a good example for children by eating fruit every day with meals or as snacks.

•Offer children a choice of fruits for lunch.

•Depending on their age, children can help shop for, clean, peel, or cut up fruits.

•While shopping, allow children to pick out a new fruit to try later at home.

•Decorate plates or serving dishes with fruit slices.

•Top off a bowl of cereal with some berries. Or, make a smiley face with sliced bananas for eyes, raisins for a nose, and an orange slice for a mouth.

•Offer raisins or other dried fruits instead of candy.

•Make fruit kabobs using pineapple chunks, bananas, grapes, and berries.

•Pack a juice box (100% juice) in children's lunches instead of soda or other sugar-sweetened beverages.

•Look for and choose fruit options, such as sliced apples,

mixed fruit cup, or 100% fruit juice in fast food restaurants.

•Offer fruit pieces and 100% fruit juice to children. There is often little fruit in "fruit-flavored" beverages or chewy fruit snacks.

Keep it safe:

•Rinse fruits before preparing or eating them. Under clean, running water, rub fruits briskly with your hands to remove dirt and surface microorganisms. Dry with a clean cloth towel or paper towel after rinsing.

•Keep fruits separate from raw meat, poultry and seafood while shopping, preparing, or storing.

<u>VEGETABLES</u>

What foods are in the Vegetable Group?

Any vegetable or 100% vegetable juice counts as a member of the Vegetable Group. Vegetables may be raw or cooked; fresh, frozen, canned, or dried/dehydrated; and may be whole, cut-up, or mashed.

Based on their nutrient content, vegetables are organized into 5 subgroups: dark-green vegetables, starchy vegetables, red and orange vegetables, beans and peas, and other vegetables.

How many vegetables are needed?

The amount of vegetables you need to eat depends on your age, sex, and level of physical activity. Recommended total daily amounts and recommended weekly amounts from each vegetable subgroup are shown in the the two charts below.

Daily Recommendation*		
Children	2-3 years old	1 cup
	4-8 years old	1 1/2 cups
Girls	9-13 years old	2 cups
	14-18 years old	2 1/2 cups

Daily Recommendation*		
Boys	9-13 years old	2 1/2 cups
	14-18 years old	3 cups
Women	19-30 years old	2 1/2 cups
	31-50 years old	2 1/2 cups
	51+ years old	2 cups
Men	19-30 years old	3 cups
	31-50 years old	3 cups
	51+ years old	2 1/2 cups

*These amounts are appropriate for individuals who get less than 30 minutes per day of moderate physical activity, beyond normal daily activities. Those who are more physically active may be able to consume more while staying within calorie needs.

Vegetable subgroup recommendations are given as amounts to eat WEEKLY. It is not necessary to eat vegetables from each subgroup daily. However, over a week, try to consume the amounts listed from each subgroup as a way to reach your daily intake recommendations.

Weekly Vegetable Subgroup Chart

	Dark green vegetables	Red and orange vegetables	Beans and peas	Starchy vegetables	Other vegetables
	Amount per Week				
Children					
2-3 yrs old	1/2 cup	2 1/2 cups	1/2 cup	2 cups	1 1/2 cups
4-8 yrs old	1 cup	3 cups	1/2 cup	3 1/2 cups	2 1/2 cups
Girls					
9-13 yrs old	1 1/2 cups	4 cups	1 cup	4 cups	3 1/2 cups
14-18 yrs old	1 1/2 cups	5 1/2 cups	1 1/2 cups	5 cups	4 cups
Boys					
9-13 yrs old	1 1/2 cups	5 1/2 cups	1 1/2 cups	5 cups	4 cups
14-18 yrs old	2 cups	6 cups	2 cups	6 cups	5 cups
Women					
19-30			1 1/2		

yrs old	1 1/2 cups	5 1/2 cups	cups	5 cups	4 cups
31-50 yrs old	1 1/2 cups	5 1/2 cups	1 1/2 cups	5 cups	4 cups
51+ yrs old	1 1/2 cups	4 cups	1 cup	4 cups	3 1/2 cups
Men					
19-30 yrs old	2 cups	6 cups	2 cups	6 cups	5 cups
31-50 yrs old	2 cups	6 cups	2 cups	6 cups	5 cups
51+ yrs old	1 1/2 cups	5 1/2 cups	1 1/2 cups	5 cups	4 cups

What counts as a cup of vegetables?

In general, 1 cup of raw or cooked vegetables or vegetable juice, or 2 cups of raw leafy greens can be considered as 1 cup from the Vegetable Group. The chart below lists specific amounts that count as 1 cup of vegetables (in some cases equivalents for ½ cup are also shown) towards your recommended intake.

Cup of Vegetable Chart		
	Amount that counts as 1 cup of vegetable	Amount that counts as 1/2 cup of vegetables
Dark Green Vegetables		
Broccoli	1 cup chopped or florets 3 spears 5" long raw or cooked	
Greens (collards, mustard greens, turnip greens, kale)	1 cup cooked	
Spinach	1 cup, cooked 2 cups raw is equivalent to 1 cup of vegetables	1 cup raw is equivalent to 1/2 cup of vegetables
Raw leafy greens: Spinach, romaine, watercress, dark green leafy lettuce,	2 cups raw is equivalent to 1 cup of vegetables	1 cup raw is equivalent to 1/2 cup of vegetables

Cup of Vegetable Chart		
	Amount that counts as 1 cup of vegetable	Amount that counts as 1/2 cup of vegetables
endive, escarole		
Red and Orange Vegetables		
Carrots	1 cup, strips, slices, or chopped, raw or cooked 2 medium 1 cup baby carrots (about 12)	1 medium carrot About 6 baby carrots
Pumpkin	1 cup mashed, cooked	
Red peppers	1 cup chopped, raw, or cooked 1 large pepper (3" diameter, 3 3/4" long)	1 small pepper
Tomatoes	1 large raw whole (3") 1 cup chopped or sliced, raw, canned, or cooked	1 small raw whole (2 1/4" diameter) 1 medium canned
Tomato juice	1 cup	1/2 cup
Sweet potato	1 large baked (2 1/4" or more diameter) 1 cup sliced or mashed, cooked	

Cup of Vegetable Chart		
	Amount that counts as 1 cup of vegetable	Amount that counts as 1/2 cup of vegetables
Winter squash (acorn, butternut, hubbard)	1 cup cubed, cooked	1/2 acorn squash, baked = 3/4 cup
Beans and Peas		
Dry beans and peas (such as black, garbanzo, kidney, pinto, or soy beans, or black eyed peas or split peas)	1 cup whole or mashed, cooked	
Starchy Vegetables		
Corn, yellow or white	1 cup 1 large ear (8" to 9" long)	1 small ear (about 6" long)
Green peas	1 cup	
White potatoes	1 cup diced, mashed 1 medium boiled or baked potato (2 1/2" to 3" diameter)	

Cup of Vegetable Chart		
	Amount that counts as 1 cup of vegetable	Amount that counts as 1/2 cup of vegetables
	French fried: 20 medium to long strips (2 1/2" to 4" long) (Contains added calories from solid fats.)	
	Amount that counts as 1 cup of vegetables	Amount that counts as 1/2 cup of vegetables
Other Vegetables		
Bean sprouts	1 cup cooked	
Cabbage, green	1 cup, chopped or shredded raw or cooked	
Cauliflower	1 cup pieces or florets raw or cooked	
Celery	1 cup, diced or sliced, raw or cooked 2 large stalks (11" to 12" long)	1 large stalk (11" to 12" long)
Cucumbers	1 cup raw, sliced or chopped	
Green or wax	1 cup cooked	

Cup of Vegetable Chart		
	Amount that counts as 1 cup of vegetable	Amount that counts as 1/2 cup of vegetables
beans		
Green peppers	1 cup chopped, raw or cooked 1 large pepper (3" diameter, 3 3/4" long)	1 small pepper
Lettuce, iceberg or head	2 cups raw, shredded or chopped = equivalent to 1 cup of vegetables	1 cup raw, shredded or chopped = equivalent to 1/2 cup of vegetables
Mushrooms	1 cup raw or cooked	
Onions	1 cup chopped, raw or cooked	
Summer squash or zucchini	1 cup cooked, sliced or diced	

Why is it important to eat vegetables?

Eating vegetables provides health benefits – people who eat more vegetables and fruits as part of an overall healthy diet are likely to have a reduced risk of some chronic diseases. Vegetables provide nutrients vital for health and maintenance of your body.

Nutrients

•Most vegetables are naturally low in fat and calories. None have cholesterol. (Sauces or seasonings may add fat, calories, and/or cholesterol.)

•Vegetables are important sources of many nutrients, including potassium, dietary fiber, folate (folic acid), vitamin A, and vitamin C.

•Diets rich in potassium may help to maintain healthy blood pressure. Vegetable sources of potassium include sweet potatoes, white potatoes, white beans, tomato products (paste, sauce, and juice), beet greens, soybeans, lima beans, spinach, lentils, and kidney beans.

•Dietary fiber from vegetables, as part of an overall healthy diet, helps reduce blood cholesterol levels and may lower risk of heart disease. Fiber is important for proper bowel function. It helps reduce constipation and diverticulosis. Fiber-containing foods such as vegetables help provide a feeling of fullness with fewer calories.

•Folate (folic acid) helps the body form red blood cells. Women of childbearing age who may become pregnant should consume adequate folate from foods, and in addition 400 mcg of synthetic folic acid from fortified foods or supplements. This reduces the risk of neural tube defects, spina bifida, and anencephaly during fetal development.

•Vitamin A keeps eyes and skin healthy and helps to protect against infections.
•Vitamin C helps heal cuts and wounds and keeps teeth and gums healthy. Vitamin C aids in iron absorption.

Health benefits

•Eating a diet rich in vegetables and fruits as part of an overall healthy diet may reduce risk for heart disease, including heart attack and stroke.
•Eating a diet rich in some vegetables and fruits as part of an overall healthy diet may protect against certain types of cancers.
•Diets rich in foods containing fiber, such as some vegetables and fruits, may reduce the risk of heart disease, obesity, and type 2 diabetes.
•Eating vegetables and fruits rich in potassium as part of an overall healthy diet may lower blood pressure, and may also reduce the risk of developing kidney stones and help to decrease bone loss.
•Eating foods such as vegetables that are lower in calories per cup instead of some other higher-calorie food may be useful in helping to lower calorie intake.

Tips to help you eat vegetables

In general:
•Buy fresh vegetables in season. They cost less and are likely to be at their peak flavor.
•Stock up on frozen vegetables for quick and easy cooking in the microwave.

•Buy vegetables that are easy to prepare. Pick up pre-washed bags of salad greens and add baby carrots or grape tomatoes for a salad in minutes. Buy packages of veggies such as baby carrots or celery sticks for quick snacks.

•Use a microwave to quickly "zap" vegetables. White or sweet potatoes can be baked quickly this way.

•Vary your veggie choices to keep meals interesting.

•Try crunchy vegetables, raw or lightly steamed.

For the best nutritional value:

•Select vegetables with more potassium often, such as sweet potatoes, white potatoes, white beans, tomato products (paste, sauce, and juice), beet greens, soybeans, lima beans, spinach, lentils, and kidney beans.

•Sauces or seasonings can add calories, saturated fat, and sodium to vegetables. Use the Nutrition Facts label to compare the calories and % Daily Value for saturated fat and sodium in plain and seasoned vegetables.

•Prepare more foods from fresh ingredients to lower sodium intake. Most sodium in the food supply comes from packaged or processed foods.

•Buy canned vegetables labeled "reduced sodium," "low sodium," or "no salt added." If you want to add a little salt it will likely be less than the amount in the regular canned product.

At meals:

•Plan some meals around a vegetable main dish, such as a vegetable stir-fry or soup. Then add other foods to complement it.

•Try a main dish salad for lunch. Go light on the salad dressing.
•Include a green salad with your dinner every night.
•Shred carrots or zucchini into meatloaf, casseroles, quick breads, and muffins.
•Include chopped vegetables in pasta sauce or lasagna.
•Order a veggie pizza with toppings like mushrooms, green peppers, and onions, and ask for extra veggies.
•Use pureed, cooked vegetables such as potatoes to thicken stews, soups and gravies. These add flavor, nutrients, and texture.
•Grill vegetable kabobs as part of a barbecue meal. Try tomatoes, mushrooms, green peppers, and onions.

Make vegetables more appealing:
•Many vegetables taste great with a dip or dressing. Try a low-fat salad dressing with raw broccoli, red and green peppers, celery sticks or cauliflower.
•Add color to salads by adding baby carrots, shredded red cabbage, or spinach leaves. Include in-season vegetables for variety through the year.
•Include beans or peas in flavorful mixed dishes, such as chili or minestrone soup.
•Decorate plates or serving dishes with vegetable slices.
•Keep a bowl of cut-up vegetables in a see-through container in the refrigerator. Carrot and celery sticks are traditional, but consider red or green pepper strips, broccoli florets, or cucumber slices.

Vegetable tips for children:

•Set a good example for children by eating vegetables with meals and as snacks.
•Let children decide on the dinner vegetables or what goes into salads.
•Depending on their age, children can help shop for, clean, peel, or cut up vegetables.
•Allow children to pick a new vegetable to try while shopping.
•Use cut-up vegetables as part of afternoon snacks.
•Children often prefer foods served separately. So, rather than mixed vegetables try serving two vegetables separately.

Keep it safe:
•Rinse vegetables before preparing or eating them. Under clean, running water, rub vegetables briskly with your hands to remove dirt and surface microorganisms. Dry with a clean cloth towel or paper towel after rinsing.
•Keep vegetables separate from raw meat, poultry and seafood while shopping, preparing, or storing.

Beans and peas are unique foods

Beans and peas are the mature forms of legumes. They include kidney beans, pinto beans, black beans, lima beans, black-eyed peas, garbanzo beans (chickpeas), split peas and lentils. They are available in dry, canned, and frozen forms. These foods are excellent sources of plant protein, and also provide other nutrients such as iron and zinc. They are similar to meats, poultry, and fish in their contribution of these nutrients. Therefore, they are considered part of the Protein Foods Group. Many people consider beans and peas as vegetarian alternatives for meat. However, they are also considered part of the Vegetable Group because they are excellent sources of dietary fiber and nutrients such as folate and potassium. These nutrients, which are often low in the diet of many Americans, are also found in other vegetables.

Because of their high nutrient content, consuming beans and peas is recommended for everyone, including people who also eat meat, poultry, and fish regularly. The USDA Food Patterns classify beans and peas as a subgroup of the Vegetable Group. The USDA Food Patterns also indicate that beans and peas may be counted as part of the Protein Foods Group. Individuals can count beans and peas as either a vegetable or a protein food.

Green peas, green lima beans, and green (string) beans are not considered to be part of the beans and peas subgroup. Green peas and green lima beans are similar to other starchy vegetables and are grouped with them. Green beans are grouped with other vegetables such as onions, lettuce, celery, and cabbage because their nutrient content is similar to those foods.

How to count beans and peas in the USDA food patterns:

Generally, individuals who regularly eat meat, poultry, and fish would count beans and peas in the Vegetable Group. Vegetarians, vegans, and individuals who seldom eat meat, poultry, or fish would count some of the beans and peas they eat in the Protein Foods Group. Here's an example for both ways:

Count the number of ounce-equivalents of all meat, poultry, fish, eggs, nuts, and seeds eaten.

1. If the total is equal to or more than the suggested intake from the Protein Foods Group (which ranges from 2 ounce-equivalents at 1,000 calories to 7 ounce-equivalents at 2,800 calories and above) then count any beans or peas eaten as part of the beans and peas subgroup in the Vegetable Group.

OR

2. If the total is less than the suggested intake from the Protein Foods Group, then count any beans and peas eaten toward the suggested intake level until it is reached. (One-fourth cup of cooked beans or peas counts as 1 ounce equivalent in the Protein Foods Group.) After the suggested intake level in the Protein Foods Group is reached, count any additional beans or peas eaten as part of the beans and peas subgroup in the Vegetable Group.

Example 1: (For the 2,000-calorie food pattern)

Foods eaten (Protein Foods Group only – not a complete daily list)
- 3½ ounces chicken
- 2 ounces tuna fish
- ½ cup refried beans

The 3½ ounces of chicken and 2 ounces of tuna fish equal 5½ ounce-equivalents in the Protein Foods Group, which meets the recommendation at this calorie level. Therefore, the ½ cup of refried beans counts as ½ cup of vegetables towards meeting the 1½ cups per week recommendation for beans and peas in the 2,000-calorie pattern.

Example 2: (For the 2,000-calorie food pattern)

Foods eaten (Protein Foods Group only – not a complete daily list)
- 2 eggs
- 1½ Tbsp. peanut butter
- ½ cup chickpeas

The 2 eggs and 1½ Tbsp. peanut butter equal 3½ ounce-equivalents in the Protein Foods Group. Two more ounces are needed to meet the 5½ ounce recommendation for this group. Since the daily recommendation for the Protein Foods Group has not been met, these remaining 2 ounce-equivalents are provided by the ½ cup of chickpeas. This ½ cup of chickpeas would not count toward meeting the 1½ cups per week recommendation for the beans and peas vegetable subgroup in the 2,000-calorie pattern. Instead, it would count as part of the Protein Foods Group.

GRAINS

What foods are in the Grains Group?

Any food made from wheat, rice, oats, cornmeal, barley or another cereal grain is a grain product. Bread, pasta, oatmeal, breakfast cereals, tortillas, and grits are examples of grain products.

Grains are divided into 2 subgroups, Whole Grains and Refined Grains. Whole grains contain the entire grain kernel — the bran, germ, and endosperm. Examples of whole grains include whole-wheat flour, bulgur (cracked wheat), oatmeal, whole cornmeal, and brown rice. Refined grains have been milled, a process that removes the bran and germ. This is done to give grains a finer texture and improve their shelf life, but it also removes dietary fiber, iron, and many B vitamins. *Some examples of refined grain products* are white flour, de-germed cornmeal, white bread, and white rice.

Most refined grains are enriched. This means certain B vitamins (thiamin, riboflavin, niacin, folic acid) and iron are added back after processing. Fiber is not added back to enriched grains. Check the ingredient list on refined grain products to make sure that the word "enriched" is included in the grain name. Some food products are made from mixtures of whole grains and refined grains.

How many grain foods are needed daily?

The amount of grains you need to eat depends on your age, sex, and level of physical activity. Recommended daily amounts are listed in this chart below. Most Americans consume enough grains, but few are whole grains. At least half of all the grains eaten should be whole grains.

Daily Grain Chart			
		DAILY RECOMMENDATION*	Daily minimum amount of whole grains
Children	2-3 years old	3 ounce equivalents	1 1/2 ounce equivalents
	4-8 years old	5 ounce equivalents	2 1/2 ounce equivalents
Girls	9-13 years old	5 ounce equivalents	3 ounce equivalents
	14-18 years old	6 ounce equivalents	3 ounce equivalents

Daily Grain Chart			
		DAILY RECOMMENDATION*	Daily minimum amount of whole grains
Boys	9-13 years old	6 ounce equivalents	3 ounce equivalents
	14-18 years old	8 ounce equivalents	4 ounce equivalents
Women	19-30 years old	6 ounce equivalents	3 ounce equivalents
	31-50 years old	6 ounce equivalents	3 ounce equivalents
	51+ years old	5 ounce equivalents	3 ounce equivalents
Men	19-30 years old	8 ounce equivalents	4 ounce equivalents
	31-50 years old	7 ounce equivalents	3 1/2 ounce equivalents
	51+ years old	6 ounce equivalents	3 ounce equivalents

*These amounts are appropriate for individuals who get less than 30 minutes per day of moderate physical activity, beyond normal daily activities. Those who are more physically active may be able to consume more while staying within calorie needs.

What counts as an ounce equivalent of grains?

In general, 1 slice of bread, 1 cup of ready-to-eat cereal, or ½ cup of cooked rice, cooked pasta, or cooked cereal can be considered as 1 ounce equivalent from the Grains Group. The chart below lists specific amounts that count as 1 ounce equivalent of grains towards your daily recommended intake. In some cases the number of ounce-equivalents for common portions are also shown.

Ounce-equivalent of grains chart			
		Amount that counts as 1 ounce equivalent of grains	Common portions and ounce equivalents
Bagels	WG**: whole wheat RG**: plain, egg	1" mini bagel	1 large bagel = 4 ounce equivalents
Biscuits	(baking powder/ buttermilk - RG*)	1 small (2" diameter)	1 large (3" diameter) = 2 ounce-equivalents
Breads	WG**: 100% Whole Wheat RG**: white, wheat, French, sourdough	1 regular slice 1 small slice French 4 snack-size slices rye bread	2 regular slices = 2 ounce-equivalents

Ounce-equivalent of grains chart			
		Amount that counts as 1 ounce equivalent of grains	Common portions and ounce equivalents
Bulgur	cracked wheat (WG**)	1/2 cup cooked	
Cornbread	(RG**)	1 small piece (2 ½" x 1 ¼" x 1¼")	1 medium piece (2 ½" x 2 ½" x 1 ¼") = 2ounce-equivalents
Crackers	WG**: 100% whole wheat, rye RG**: saltines, snack crackers	5 whole wheat crackers 2 rye crispbreads 7 square or round crackers	
English muffins	WG**: whole wheat RG**: plain, raisin	½ muffin	1 muffin = 2 ounce equivalents
Muffins	WG**: whole wheat	1 small (2 ½" diameter)	1 large (3 ½" diameter) = 3 ounce

Ounce-equivalent of grains chart			
		Amount that counts as 1 ounce equivalent of grains	Common portions and ounce equivalents
	RG**: bran, corn, plain		equivalents
Oatmeal	(WG**)	½ cup cooked 1 packet instant 1 ounce (1/3 cup) dry (regular or quick)	
Pancakes	WG**: Whole wheat, buckwheat RG**: buttermilk, plain	1 pancake (4 ½" diameter) 2 small pancakes (3" diameter)	3 pancakes (4 ½" diameter) = 3 ounce-equivalents
Popcorn	(WG**)	3 cups, popped	1 mini microwave bag or 100-calorie bag, popped =2 ounce-equivalents
Ready-to eat	WG**: toasted	1 cup flakes or rounds	

Ounce-equivalent of grains chart			
		Amount that counts as 1 ounce equivalent of grains	Common portions and ounce equivalents
breakfast cereal	oat, whole wheat flakes RG**: corn flakes, puffed rice	1 ¼ cup puffed	
Rice	WG*: brown, wild RG*: enriched, white, polished	½ cup cooked 1 ounce dry	1 cup cooked = 2 ounce-equivalents
Pasta-- spaghetti, macaroni, noodles	WG**: whole wheat RG**: enriched, durum	½ cup cooked 1 ounce dry	1 cup cooked = 2 ounce-equivalents
Tortillas	WG**: whole wheat, whole grain corn	1 small flour tortilla (6" diameter) 1 corn tortilla (6" diameter)	1 large tortilla (12" diameter) = 4 ounce equivalents

Ounce-equivalent of grains chart			
		Amount that counts as 1 ounce equivalent of grains	Common portions and ounce equivalents
	RG**: Flour, corn		

*WG = whole grains, RG = refined grains. This is shown when products are available both in whole grain and refined grain forms.

Why is it important to eat grains, especially whole grains?

Eating grains, especially whole grains, provides health benefits. People who eat whole grains as part of a healthy diet have a reduced risk of some chronic diseases. Grains provide many nutrients that are vital for the health and maintenance of our bodies.

•Grains are important sources of many nutrients, including dietary fiber, several B vitamins (thiamin, riboflavin, niacin, and folate), and minerals (iron, magnesium, and selenium).

•Dietary fiber from whole grains or other foods, may help reduce blood cholesterol levels and may lower risk of heart disease, obesity, and type 2 diabetes. Fiber is important for proper bowel function. It helps reduce constipation and diverticulosis. Fiber-containing foods such as whole grains help provide a feeling of fullness with fewer calories.

•The B vitamins thiamin, riboflavin, and niacin play a key role in metabolism – they help the body release energy from protein, fat, and carbohydrates. B vitamins are also essential for a healthy nervous system. Many refined grains are enriched with these B vitamins.

•Folate (folic acid), another B vitamin, helps the body form red blood cells. Women of childbearing age who may become pregnant should consume adequate folate from foods, and in addition 400 mcg of synthetic folic acid from fortified foods or supplements. This reduces the risk of neural tube defects, spina bifida, and anencephaly during fetal development.

•Iron is used to carry oxygen in the blood. Many teenage girls and women in their childbearing years have iron-deficiency anemia. They should eat foods high in heme-iron (meats) or eat other iron containing foods along with foods rich in vitamin C, which can improve absorption of non-heme iron. Whole and enriched refined grain products are major sources of non-heme iron in American diets.

•Whole grains are sources of magnesium and selenium. Magnesium is a mineral used in building bones and releasing energy from muscles. Selenium protects cells from oxidation. It is also important for a healthy immune system.

Health benefits

•Consuming whole grains as part of a healthy diet may reduce the risk of heart disease.

•Consuming foods containing fiber, such as whole grains, as part of a healthy diet, may reduce constipation.

•Eating whole grains may help with weight management.

•Eating grain products fortified with folate before and during pregnancy helps prevent neural tube defects during fetal development.

Tips to help you eat whole grains

At meals:

- To eat more whole grains, substitute a whole-grain product for a refined product – such as eating whole-wheat bread instead of white bread or brown rice instead of white rice. It's important to *substitute* the whole-grain product for the refined one, rather than *adding* the whole-grain product.
- For a change, try brown rice or whole-wheat pasta. Try brown rice stuffing in baked green

peppers or tomatoes and whole-wheat macaroni in macaroni and cheese.

- Use whole grains in mixed dishes, such as barley in vegetable soup or stews and bulgur wheat in a casserole or stir-fry.
- Create a whole grain pilaf with a mixture of barley, wild rice, brown rice, broth and spices. For a special touch, stir in toasted nuts or chopped dried fruit.
- Experiment by substituting whole wheat or oat flour for up to half of the flour in pancake, waffle, muffin or other flour-based recipes. They may need a bit more leavening.
- Use whole-grain bread or cracker crumbs in meatloaf.
- Try rolled oats or a crushed, unsweetened whole grain cereal as breading for baked chicken, fish, veal cutlets, or eggplant parmesan.
- Try an unsweetened, whole grain ready-to-eat cereal as croutons in salad or in place of crackers with soup.
- Freeze leftover cooked brown rice, bulgur, or barley. Heat and serve it later as a quick side dish.

As snacks:

- Snack on ready-to-eat, whole grain cereals such as toasted oat cereal.

- Add whole-grain flour or oatmeal when making cookies or other baked treats.
- Try 100% whole-grain snack crackers.
- Popcorn, a whole grain, can be a healthy snack if made with little or no added salt and butter.

What to look for on the food label:

- Choose foods that name one of the following whole-grain ingredients first on the label's ingredient list:

Whole grain ingredients

- brown rice
- buckwheat
- bulgur
- millet
- oatmeal
- popcorn
- quinoa
- rolled oats

- whole-grain barley
- whole-grain corn
- whole-grain sorghum
- whole-grain triticale
- whole oats
- whole rye
- whole wheat
- wild rice

- Foods labeled with the words "multi-grain," "stone-ground," "100% wheat," "cracked wheat," "seven-grain," or "bran" are usually not whole-grain products.

- Color is not an indication of a whole grain. Bread can be brown because of molasses or other added ingredients. Read the ingredient list to see if it is a whole grain.
- Use the Nutrition Facts label and choose whole grain products with a higher % Daily Value (% DV) for fiber. Many, but not all, whole grain products are good or excellent sources of fiber.
- Read the food label's ingredient list. Look for terms that indicate added sugars (such as sucrose, high-fructose corn syrup, honey, malt syrup, maple syrup, molasses, or raw sugar) that add extra calories. Choose foods with fewer added sugars.
- Most sodium in the food supply comes from packaged foods. Similar packaged foods can vary widely in sodium content, including breads. Use the Nutrition Facts label to choose foods with a lower % DV for sodium. Foods with less than 140 mg sodium per serving can be labeled as low sodium foods. Claims such as "low in sodium" or "very low in sodium" on the front of the food label can help you identify foods that contain less salt (or sodium).

Whole grain tips for children

- Set a good example for children by eating whole grains with meals or as snacks.

- Let children select and help prepare a whole grain side dish.
- Teach older children to read the ingredient list on cereals or snack food packages and choose those with whole grains at the top of the list.

PROTEINS

What foods are in the Protein Foods Group?

All foods made from meat, poultry, seafood, beans and peas, eggs, processed soy products, nuts, and seeds are considered part of the Protein Foods Group. Beans and peas are also part of the Vegetable Group. For more information on beans and peas, see Beans and Peas Are Unique Foods.

Select a variety of protein foods to improve nutrient intake and health benefits, including at least 8 ounces of cooked seafood per week. Young children need less, depending on their age and calorie needs. The advice to consume seafood does not apply to vegetarians. Vegetarian options in the Protein Foods Group include beans and peas, processed soy products, and nuts and seeds. Meat and poultry choices should be lean or low-fat.

How much food from the Protein Foods Group is daily?

The amount of food from the Protein Foods Group you need to eat depends on age, sex, and level of physical activity. Most Americans eat enough food from this group, but need to make leaner and more varied selections of these foods. Recommended daily amounts are shown in the chart below.

Daily protein foods chart		
Daily recommendation*		
Children	2-3 years old	2 ounce equivalents
	4-8 years old	4 ounce equivalents
Girls	9-13 years old	5 ounce equivalents
	14-18 years old	5 ounce equivalents
Boys	9-13 years old	5 ounce equivalents
	14-18 years old	6 1/2 ounce equivalents
Women	19-30 years old	5 1/2 ounce equivalents
	31-50 years old	5 ounce equivalents
	51+ years old	5 ounce equivalents
Men	19-30 years old	6 1/2 ounce equivalents
	31-50 years old	6 ounce equivalents
	51+ years old	5 1/2 ounce equivalents

*These amounts are appropriate for individuals who get less than 30 minutes per day of moderate physical activity, beyond normal daily activities. Those who are more physically active may be able to consume more while staying within calorie needs.

What counts as an ounce-equivalent in the Protein Foods Group?

In general, 1 ounce of meat, poultry or fish, ¼ cup cooked beans, 1 egg, 1 tablespoon of peanut butter, or ½ ounce of nuts or seeds can be considered as 1 ounce-equivalent from the Protein Foods Group.

This chart below lists specific amounts that count as 1 ounce-equivalent in the Protein Foods Group towards your daily recommended intake.

ounce-equivalent of protein foods chart		
	Amount that counts as 1 ounce-equivalent in the Protein Foods Group	Common portions and ounce-equivalents
Meats	1 ounce cooked lean beef 1 ounce cooked lean pork or ham	1 small steak (eye of round, filet) = 3 1/2 to 4 ounce-equivalents 1 small lean hamburger = 2 to 3 ounce-equivalents
Poultry	1 ounce cooked chicken or turkey, without skin 1 sandwich slice of turkey (4 1/2" x 2 1/2" x 1/8")	1 small chicken breast half = 3 ounce-equivalents 1/2 Cornish game hen = 4 ounce-equivalents
Seafood	1 ounce cooked fish or shell fish	1 can of tuna, drained = 3 to 4 ounce-

ounce-equivalent of protein foods chart		
	Amount that counts as 1 ounce-equivalent in the Protein Foods Group	Common portions and ounce-equivalents
		equivalents 1 salmon steak = 4 to 6 ounce-equivalents 1 small trout = 3 ounce-equivalents
Eggs	1 egg	3 egg whites = 2 ounce-equivalents 3 egg yolks = 1 ounce-equivalent
Nuts and seeds	1/2 ounce of nuts (12 almonds, 24 pistachios, 7 walnut halves) 1/2 ounce of seeds (pumpkin, sunflower, or squash seeds, hulled, roasted) 1 Tablespoon of peanut butter or almond butter	1 ounce of nuts of seeds = 2 ounce-equivalents
Beans and peas	1/4 cup of cooked beans (such as black, kidney, pinto, or white beans) 1/4 cup of cooked peas (such as chickpeas, cowpeas, lentils, or split peas) 1/4 cup of baked beans,	1 cup split pea soup = 2 ounce-equivalents 1 cup lentil soup = 2 ounce-equivalents 1 cup bean soup = 2 ounce-equivalents

ounce-equivalent of protein foods chart		
	Amount that counts as 1 ounce-equivalent in the Protein Foods Group	Common portions and ounce-equivalents
	refried beans 1/4 cup (about 2 ounces) of tofu 1 ox. tempeh, cooked 1/4 cup roasted soybeans 1 falafel patty (2 1/4", 4 oz) 2 Tablespoons hummus	1 soy or bean burger patty = 2 ounce-equivalents

Selection Tips

- Choose lean or low-fat meat and poultry. If higher fat choices are made, such as regular ground beef (75-80% lean) or chicken with skin, the fat counts against your maximum limit for empty calories (calories from solid fats or added sugars).
- If solid fat is added in cooking, such as frying chicken in shortening or frying eggs in butter or stick margarine, this also counts against your maximum limit for empty calories (calories from solid fats and added sugars).
- Select some seafood that is rich in omega-3 fatty acids, such as salmon, trout, sardines, anchovies, herring, Pacific oysters, and Atlantic and Pacific mackerel.

- Processed meats such as ham, sausage, frankfurters, and luncheon or deli meats have added sodium. Check the Nutrition Facts label to help limit sodium intake. Fresh chicken, turkey, and pork that have been enhanced with a salt-containing solution also have added sodium. Check the product label for statements such as "self-basting" or "contains up to __% of __", which mean that a sodium-containing solution has been added to the product.
- Choose unsalted nuts and seeds to keep sodium intake low.

Why is it important to make lean or low-fat choices from the Protein Foods Group?

Foods in the meat, poultry, fish, eggs, nuts, and seed group provide nutrients that are vital for health and maintenance of your body. However, choosing foods from this group that are high in saturated fat and cholesterol may have health implications.

The chart below lists specific amounts that count as 1 ounce equivalent in the Protein Foods Group towards your daily recommended intake:

	Amount that counts as 1 ounce equivalent in the Protein Foods Group	Common portions and ounce equivalents
Meats	1 ounce cooked lean	1 small steak (eye of round, filet) = 3/12 to

	Amount that counts as 1 ounce equivalent in the Protein Foods Group	Common portions and ounce equivalents
	beef 1 ounce cooked lean pork or ham	4 ounce equivalents 1 small lean hamburger = 2 to 3 ounce equivalents
Poultry	1 ounce cooked chicken or turkey, without skin 1 sandwich slice of turkey (4 1/2 x 2 1/2 x 1/8")	1 small chicken breast half = 3 ounce equivalents 1/2 Cornish game hen = 4 ounce equivalents
Seafood	1 ounce cooked fish or shell fish	1 can of tuna, drained = 3 to 4 ounce equivalents 1 salmon steak = 4 to 6 ounce equivalents 1 small trout = 3 ounce equivalents
Eggs	1 egg	3 egg whites = 2 ounce equivalents 3 egg yolks = 1 ounce equivalent
Nuts and seeds	1/2 ounce of nuts (12 almonds, 24 pistachios, 7 walnut halves) 1/2 ounce of seeds (pumpkin, sunflower, or squash seeds, hulled,	1 ounce of nuts of seeds = 2 ounce equivalents

	Amount that counts as 1 ounce equivalent in the Protein Foods Group	Common portions and ounce equivalents
	roasted) 1 Tablespoon of peanut butter or almond butter	
Beans and peas	1/4 cup of cooked beans (such as black, kidney, pinto, or white beans) 1/4 cup of cooked peas (such as chickpeas, cowpeas, lentils, or split peas) 1/4 cup of baked beans, refried beans	1 cup split pea soup = 2 ounce equivalents 1 cup lentil soup = 2 ounce equivalents 1 cup bean soup = 2 ounce equivalents
	1/4 cup (about 2 ounces) of tofu 1 ox. tempeh, cooked 1/4 cup roasted soybeans 1 falafel patty (2 1/4", 4 oz) 2 Tablespoons hummus	1 soy or bean burger patty = 2 ounce equivalents

Nutrients

- Diets that are high in saturated fats raise "bad" cholesterol levels in the blood. The "bad" cholesterol is called LDL (low-density lipoprotein) cholesterol. High LDL cholesterol, in turn, increases the risk for coronary heart disease.

Some food choices in this group are high in saturated fat. These include fatty cuts of beef, pork, and lamb; regular (75% to 85% lean) ground beef; regular sausages, hot dogs, and bacon; some luncheon meats such as regular bologna and salami; and some poultry such as duck. To help keep blood cholesterol levels healthy, limit the amount of these foods you eat.

- Diets that are high in cholesterol can raise LDL cholesterol levels in the blood. Cholesterol is only found in foods from animal sources. Some foods from this group are high in cholesterol. These include egg yolks (egg whites are cholesterol-free) and organ meats such as liver and giblets. To help keep blood cholesterol levels healthy, limit the amount of these foods you eat.
- A high intake of fats makes it difficult to avoid consuming more calories than are needed.

Why is it important to eat 8 ounces of seafood per week?

- Seafood contains a range of nutrients, notably the omega-3 fatty acids, EPA and DHA. Eating about 8 ounces per week of a variety of seafood contributes to the prevention of heart disease. Smaller amounts of seafood are recommended for young children.
- Seafood varieties that are commonly consumed in the United States that are higher in EPA and DHA and lower in mercury include salmon, anchovies,

herring, sardines, Pacific oysters, trout, and Atlantic and Pacific mackerel (not king mackerel, which is high in mercury). The health benefits from consuming seafood outweigh the health risk associated with mercury, a heavy metal found in seafood in varying levels.

Health benefits

- Meat, poultry, fish, dry beans and peas, eggs, nuts, and seeds supply many nutrients. These include protein, B vitamins (niacin, thiamin, riboflavin, and B6), vitamin E, iron, zinc, and magnesium.
- Proteins function as building blocks for bones, muscles, cartilage, skin, and blood. They are also building blocks for enzymes, hormones, and vitamins. Proteins are one of three nutrients that provide calories (the others are fat and carbohydrates).
- B vitamins found in this food group serve a variety of functions in the body. They help the body release energy, play a vital role in the function of the nervous system, aid in the formation of red blood cells, and help build tissues.
- Iron is used to carry oxygen in the blood. Many teenage girls and women in their child-bearing years have iron-deficiency anemia. They should eat foods high in heme-iron (meats) or eat other non-heme iron containing foods along with a food

rich in vitamin C, which can improve absorption of non-heme iron.

- Magnesium is used in building bones and in releasing energy from muscles.
- Zinc is necessary for biochemical reactions and helps the immune system function properly.
- EPA and DHA are omega-3 fatty acids found in varying amounts in seafood. Eating 8 ounces per week of seafood may help reduce the risk for heart disease.

What are the benefits of eating nuts and seeds?

- Eating peanuts and certain tree nuts (i.e., walnuts, almonds, and pistachios) may reduce the risk of heart disease when consumed as part of a diet that is nutritionally adequate and within calorie needs. Because nuts and seeds are high in calories, eat them in small portions and use them to replace other protein foods, like some meat or poultry, rather than adding them to what you already eat. In addition, choose unsalted nuts and seeds to help reduce sodium intakes.

Vegetarian choices in the Protein Foods GroupVegetarians get enough protein from this group as long as the variety and amounts of foods selected are adequate. Protein sources from the Protein Foods Group for vegetarians include eggs (for ovo-vegetarians), beans and peas, nuts, nut butters, and soy products (tofu, tempeh, veggie burgers).

Tips to help you make wise choices from the Protein Foods Group

Go lean with protein:
•The leanest beef cuts include round steaks and roasts (eye of round, top round, bottom round, round tip), top loin, top sirloin, and chuck shoulder and arm roasts.
•The leanest pork choices include pork loin, tenderloin, center loin, and ham.
•Choose lean ground beef. To be considered "lean," the product has to be at least 92% lean/8% fat.
•Buy skinless chicken parts, or take off the skin before cooking.
•Boneless skinless chicken breasts and turkey cutlets are the leanest poultry choices.
•Choose lean turkey, roast beef, ham, or low-fat luncheon meats for sandwiches instead of luncheon/deli meats with more fat, such as regular bologna or salami.

Vary your protein choices:
•Choose seafood at least twice a week as the main protein food. Look for seafood rich in omega-3 fatty acids, such as salmon, trout, and herring. Some ideas are:◦Salmon steak or filet
◦Salmon loaf
◦Grilled or baked trout

•Choose beans, peas, or soy products as a main dish or part of a meal often. Some choices are:◦Chili with kidney or pinto beans

◦Stir-fried tofu

◦Split pea, lentil, minestrone, or white bean soups

◦Baked beans

◦Black bean enchiladas

◦Garbanzo or kidney beans on a chef's salad

◦Rice and beans

◦Veggie burgers

◦Hummus (chickpeas spread) on pita bread

•Choose unsalted nuts as a snack, on salads, or in main dishes. Use nuts to replace meat or poultry, not in addition to these items:◦Use pine nuts in pesto sauce for pasta.

◦Add slivered almonds to steamed vegetables.

◦Add toasted peanuts or cashews to a vegetable stir fry instead of meat.

◦Sprinkle a few nuts on top of low-fat ice cream or frozen yogurt.

◦Add walnuts or pecans to a green salad instead of cheese or meat.

What to look for on the food label:

•Check the Nutrition Facts Label for the saturated fat, trans fat, cholesterol, and sodium content of packaged foods.◦Processed meats such as hams, sausages, frankfurters, and luncheon or deli meats have added sodium. Check the ingredient and Nutrition Facts label to help limit sodium intake.

◦Fresh chicken, turkey, and pork that have been enhanced with a salt-containing solution also have added sodium. Check the product label for statements such as "self-basting" or "contains up to __% of __."

◦Lower fat versions of many processed meats are available. Look on the Nutrition Facts label to choose products with less fat and saturated fat.

Keep it safe to eat:
- Separate raw, cooked and ready-to-eat foods.
- Do not wash or rinse meat or poultry.
- Wash cutting boards, knives, utensils and counter tops in hot soapy water after preparing each food item and before going on to the next one.
- Store raw meat, poultry and seafood on the bottom shelf of the refrigerator so juices don't drip onto other foods.
- Cook foods to a safe temperature to kill microorganisms. Use a meat thermometer, which measures the internal temperature of cooked meat and poultry, to make sure that the meat is cooked all the way through.
- Chill (refrigerate) perishable food promptly and defrost foods properly. Refrigerate or freeze perishables, prepared food and leftovers within two hours.
- Plan ahead to defrost foods. Never defrost food on the kitchen counter at room temperature. Thaw food by placing it in the refrigerator, submerging air-tight packaged food in cold tap water (change water every 30 minutes), or defrosting on a plate in the microwave.

•Avoid raw or partially cooked eggs or foods containing raw eggs and raw or undercooked meat and poultry.
•Women who may become pregnant, pregnant women, nursing mothers, and young children should avoid some types of fish and eat types lower in mercury.

DAIRY

What foods are included in the Dairy Group?

All fluid milk products and many foods made from milk are considered part of this food group. Most Dairy Group choices should be fat-free or low-fat. Foods made from milk that retain their calcium content are part of the group. Foods made from milk that have little to no calcium, such as cream cheese, cream, and butter, are not. Calcium-fortified soymilk (soy beverage) is also part of the Dairy Group.

How much food from the Dairy Group is needed daily?

The amount of food from the Dairy Group you need to eat depends on age. Recommended daily amounts are shown in the chart below.

Daily Dairy Chart					
Daily recommendation					
Children	2-3 years old	2 cups	Women	19-30 years old	3 cups
	4-8 years old	2 ½ cups		31-50 years old	3 cups
Girls	9-13 years old	3 cups		51+ years old	3 cups
	14-18 years old	3 cups	Men	19-30 years old	3 cups
Boys	9-13 years old	3 cups		31-50 years old	3 cups
	14-18 years old	3 cups		51+ years old	3 cups

What counts as a cup in the Dairy Group?

In general, 1 cup of milk, yogurt, or soymilk (soy beverage), 1 ½ ounces of natural cheese, or 2 ounces of processed cheese can be considered as 1 cup from the Dairy Group. The chart below lists specific amounts that count as 1 cup in the Dairy Group towards your daily recommended intake.

Cup of dairy chart		
	Amount That Counts as a Cup in the Dairy Group	Common Portions and Cup Equivalents
Milk (choose fat-free or low-fat milk)	1 cup milk	
	1 half-pint container milk	
	½ cup evaporated milk	
Yogurt (choose fat-free or low-fat yogurt)	1 regular container (8 fluid ounces)	1 small container (6 ounces) = ¾ cup
	1 cup yogurt	1 snack size container (4 ounces) = ½ cup
Cheese (choose reduced-fat or low-fat cheeses)	1 ½ ounces hard cheese (cheddar, mozzarella, Swiss, Parmesan)	1 slice of hard cheese is equivalent to ½ cup milk
	⅓ cup shredded cheese	
	2 ounces processed	1 slice of processed

Cup of dairy chart		
	Amount That Counts as a Cup in the Dairy Group	Common Portions and Cup Equivalents
	cheese (American)	cheese is equivalent to ⅓ cup milk
	½ cup ricotta cheese	
	2 cups cottage cheese	½ cup cottage cheese is equivalent to ¼ cup milk
Milk-based desserts (choose fat-free or low-fat types)	1 cup pudding made with milk	
	1 cup frozen yogurt	
	1 ½ cups ice cream	1 scoop ice cream is equivalent to ⅓ cup milk
Soymilk (soy beverage)	1 cup calcium-fortified soymilk	
	1 half-pint container calcium-fortified soymilk	

Selection tips

- Choose fat-free or low-fat milk, yogurt, and cheese. If you choose milk or yogurt that is not fat-free, or cheese that is not low-fat, the fat in the product counts against your maximum limit for "empty calories" (calories from solid fats and added sugars).

- If sweetened milk products are chosen (flavored milk, yogurt, drinkable yogurt, desserts), the added sugars also count against your maximum limit for "empty calories" (calories from solid fats and added sugars).
- For those who are lactose intolerant, smaller portions (such as 4 fluid ounces of milk) may be well tolerated. Lactose-free and lower-lactose products are available. These include lactose-reduced or lactose-free milk, yogurt, and cheese, and calcium-fortified soymilk (soy beverage). Also, enzyme preparations can be added to milk to lower the lactose content.
- Calcium choices for those who do not consume dairy products include: kale leaves
    - Calcium-fortified juices, cereals, breads, rice milk, or almond milk. Calcium-fortified foods and beverages may not provide the other nutrients found in dairy products. Check the labels.
    - Canned fish (sardines, salmon with bones) soybeans and other soy products (tofu made with calcium sulfate, soy yogurt, tempeh), some other beans, and some leafy greens (collard and turnip greens, kale, bok choy). The amount of calcium that can be absorbed from these foods varies.

Nutrients and health benefits

Consuming dairy products provides health benefits – especially improved bone health. Foods in the Dairy Group provide nutrients that are vital for health and maintenance of your body. These nutrients include calcium, potassium, vitamin D, and protein.

Nutrients

- Calcium is used for building bones and teeth and in maintaining bone mass. Dairy products are the primary source of calcium in American diets. Diets that provide 3 cups or the equivalent of dairy products per day can improve bone mass.
- Diets rich in potassium may help to maintain healthy blood pressure. Dairy products, especially yogurt, fluid milk, and soymilk (soy beverage), provide potassium.
- Vitamin D functions in the body to maintain proper levels of calcium and phosphorous, thereby helping to build and maintain bones. Milk and soymilk (soy beverage) that are fortified with vitamin D are good sources of this nutrient. Other sources include vitamin D-fortified yogurt and vitamin D-fortified ready-to-eat breakfast cereals.
- Milk products that are consumed in their low-fat or fat-free forms provide little or no solid fat.

Health benefits

- Intake of dairy products is linked to improved bone health, and may reduce the risk of osteoporosis.
- The intake of dairy products is especially important to bone health during childhood and adolescence, when bone mass is being built.
- Intake of dairy products is also associated with a reduced risk of cardiovascular disease and type 2 diabetes, and with lower blood pressure in adults.

Why is it important to make fat-free or low-fat choices from the Dairy Group?

Choosing foods from the Dairy Group that are high in saturated fats and cholesterol can have health implications. Diets high in saturated fats raise "bad" cholesterol levels in the blood. The "bad" cholesterol is called LDL (low-density lipoprotein) cholesterol. High LDL cholesterol, in turn, increases the risk for coronary heart disease. Many cheeses, whole milk, and products made from them are high in saturated fat. To help keep blood cholesterol levels healthy, limit the amount of these foods you eat. In addition, a high intake of fats makes it difficult to avoid consuming more calories than are needed.

For those who choose not to consume milk products

Calcium choices for those who do not consume dairy products include:

- Calcium-fortified juices, cereals, breads, rice milk, or almond milk.
- Canned fish (sardines, salmon with bones) soybeans and other soy products (tofu made with calcium sulfate, soy yogurt, tempeh), some other beans, and some leafy greens (collard and turnip greens, kale, bok choy). The amount of calcium that can be absorbed from these foods varies

Tips for making wise choices in the Dairy Group

- Include milk or calcium-fortified soymilk (soy beverage) as a beverage at meals. Choose fat-free or low-fat milk.
- If you usually drink whole milk, switch gradually to fat-free milk, to lower saturated fat and calories. Try reduced fat (2%), then low-fat fruits and yogurt(1%), and finally fat-free (skim).
- If you drink cappuccinos or lattes — ask for them with fat-free (skim) milk.
- Add fat-free or low-fat milk instead of water to oatmeal and hot cereals.
- Use fat-free or low-fat milk when making condensed cream soups (such as cream of tomato).
- Have fat-free or low-fat yogurt as a snack.
- Make a dip for fruits or vegetables from yogurt.

- Make fruit-yogurt smoothies in the blender.
- For dessert, make chocolate or butterscotch pudding with fat-free or low-fat milk.
- Top cut-up fruit with flavored yogurt for a quick dessert.
- Top casseroles, soups, stews, or vegetables with shredded reduced-fat or low-fat cheese.
- Top a baked potato with fat-free or low-fat yogurt.

Keep it safe
- Avoid raw (unpasteurized) milk or any products made from unpasteurized milk.
- Chill (refrigerate) perishable food promptly and defrost foods properly. Refrigerate or freeze perishables, prepared food and leftovers as soon as possible. If food has been left at temperatures between 40° and 140° F for more than two hours, discard it, even though it may look and smell good.
- Separate raw, cooked and ready-to-eat foods.

For those who choose not to consume milk products

- If you avoid milk because of lactose intolerance, the most reliable way to get the health benefits of dairy products is to choose lactose-free alternatives within the Dairy Group, such as cheese, yogurt, lactose-free milk, or calcium-

fortified soymilk (soy beverage) — or to consume the enzyme lactase before consuming milk.
- If you avoid milk for other reasons, choose non-dairy calcium choices such as:
    - Calcium-fortified juices, cereals, breads, rice milk, almond milk, or calcium-fortified soymilk (soy beverage).
    - Canned fish (sardines, salmon with bones) soybeans and other soy products (tofu made with calcium sulfate, soy yogurt, tempeh), some other beans, and some leafy greens (collard and turnip greens, kale, bok choy). The amount of calcium that can be absorbed from these foods varies.

OILS

What are "oils"?

Oils are fats that are liquid at room temperature, like the vegetable oils used in cooking. Oils come from many different plants and from fish. Oils are NOT a food group, but they provide essential nutrients. Therefore, oils are included in USDA food patterns.

Some commonly eaten oils include: canola oil, corn oil, cottonseed oil, olive oil, safflower oil, soybean oil, and sunflower oil. Some oils are used mainly as flavorings, such as walnut oil and sesame oil. A number of foods are naturally high in oils, like nuts, olives, some fish, and avocados.

Foods that are mainly oil include mayonnaise, certain salad dressings, and soft (tub or squeeze) margarine with no trans fats. Check the Nutrition Facts label to find margarines with 0 grams of trans fat. Amounts of trans fat are required to be listed on labels.

Most oils are high in monounsaturated or polyunsaturated fats, and low in saturated fats. Oils from plant sources (vegetable and nut oils) do not contain any cholesterol. In fact, no plant foods contain cholesterol. A few plant oils, however, including coconut oil, palm oil, and palm kernel oil, are high in saturated fats and for nutritional purposes should be considered to be solid fats.

Solid fats are fats that are solid at room temperature, like butter and shortening. Solid fats come from many animal foods and can be made from vegetable oils through a process called hydrogenation. Some common fats are: butter, milk fat, beef fat (tallow, suet), chicken fat, pork fat (lard), stick margarine, shortening, and partially hydrogenated oil.

How much is my allowance for oils?

Some Americans consume enough oil in the foods they eat, such as:

- nuts
- fish

- cooking oil
- salad dressings

Others could easily consume the recommended allowance by substituting oils for some solid fats they eat. A person's allowance for oils depends on age, sex, and level of physical activity. Daily allowances for oils are shown in the chart below.

Daily Allowance		
Children	2-3 years old	3 teaspoons
	4-8 years old	4 teaspoons
Girls	9-13 years old	5 teaspoons
	14-18 years old	5 teaspoons
Boys	9-13 years old	5 teaspoons
	14-18 years old	6 teaspoons
Women	19-30 years old	6 teaspoons
	31-50 years old	5 teaspoons
	51+ years old	5 teaspoons
Men	19-30 years old	7 teaspoons
	31-50 years old	6 teaspoons
	51+ years old	6 teaspoons

How do I count the oils I eat?

The chart below gives a quick guide to the amount of oils in some common foods.

Oil Chart				
	Amount of food	Amount of oil	Calories from oil	Total calories
		Teaspoons/grams	Approximate calories	Approximate calories
Oils:				
Vegetable oils (such as canola, corn, cottonseed, olive, peanut, safflower, soybean, and sunflower)	1 Tbsp	3 tsp/14 g	120	120
Foods rich in oils:				
Margarine, soft (trans fat free)	1 Tbsp	2 ½ tsp/11 g	100	100
Mayonnaise	1 Tbsp	2 ½ tsp/11 g	100	100
Mayonnaise-type	1 Tbsp	1 tsp/5 g	45	55

Oil Chart				
	Amount of food	Amount of oil	Calories from oil	Total calories
salad dressing				
Italian dressing	2 Tbsp	2 tsp/8 g	75	85
Thousand Island dressing	2 Tbsp	2 ½ tsp/11 g	100	120
Olives*, ripe, canned	4 large	½ tsp/ 2 g	15	20
Avocado*	½ med	3 tsp/15 g	130	160
Peanut butter*	2 T	4 tsp/16 g	140	190
Peanuts, dry roasted*	1 oz	3 tsp/14 g	120	165
Mixed nuts, dry roasted*	1 oz	3 tsp/15 g	130	170
Cashews, dry roasted*	1 oz	3 tsp/13 g	115	165
Almonds, dry roasted*	1 oz	3 tsp/15 g	130	170
Hazelnuts*	1 oz	4 tsp/ 18 g	160	185

Oil Chart				
	Amount of food	Amount of oil	Calories from oil	Total calories
Sunflower seeds*	1 oz	3 tsp/ 14 g	120	165

*Avocados and olives are part of the Vegetable Group; nuts and seeds are part of the Protein Foods Group. These foods are also high in oils. Soft margarine, mayonnaise, and salad dressings are mainly oil and are not considered to be part of any food group.

How are oils different from solid fats?
All fats and oils are a mixture of saturated fatty acids and unsaturated fatty acids. Unsaturated fatty acids include *mono*unsaturated and *poly*unsaturated fats.

Oils are fats that are liquid at room temperature, like the vegetable oils used in cooking. Oils come from many different plants and from fish. Oils contain more monounsaturated and polyunsaturated fats.

Solid fats are fats that are solid at room temperature, like beef fat, butter, and shortening. Solid fats mainly come from animal foods and can also be made from vegetable oils through a process called hydrogenation. Solid fats contain more saturated fats and/or trans fats than oils. Saturated fats, trans fats, and cholesterol tend to raise "bad" (LDL) cholesterol levels in the blood, which in turn increases the risk for heart disease. To lower risk for heart disease, cut back on foods containing saturated fats, trans fats, and cholesterol.

Why is it important to consume oils?

Oils are not a food group, but they do provide essential nutrients and are therefore included in USDA recommendations for what to eat. Note that only small amounts of oils are recommended.

Most of the fats you eat should be polyunsaturated (PUFA) or monounsaturated (MUFA) fats. Oils are the major source of MUFAs and PUFAs in the diet. PUFAs contain some fatty acids that are necessary for health – called "essential fatty acids."
Because oils contain these essential fatty acids, there is an allowance for oils in the food guide.
The MUFAs and PUFAs found in fish, nuts, and vegetable oils do not raise LDL ("bad") cholesterol levels in the blood. In addition to the essential fatty acids they contain, oils are the major source of vitamin E in typical American diets.
While consuming some oil is needed for health, oils still contain calories. In fact, oils and solid fats both contain about 120 calories per tablespoon. Therefore, the amount of oil consumed needs to be limited to balance total calorie intake. The Nutrition Facts label provides information to help you make smart choices.

As you know by now the two largest groups of foodstuffs that you should be consuming are the grains and the vegetables, whilst meat products and beans are far less prominent. However, you should also make sure that when you are constructing a healthy balanced diet based on the information provided, you should be using the most nutritious alternatives possible.

For example, a significant percentage of the grain products that you eat should be whole grains such as brown rice, whereas as suggested earlier, the most nutritious vegetable and fruits are always the organic variety. Moreover, if you are including meat in your diet, it would be best to look for organic but also non.antibiotic treated meat products.

Sure, there is no doubt that if you buy the best quality food available, you will have to pay a little more but in the long run, it may even work out cheaper. If for example you can save a few hundred dollars on medical bills every year because you (and perhaps your family) are healthier than you have ever been, then the extra outlay on better quality foods is more than justified.

One final factor to bear in mind is that it is your brain that controls how energetic you feel. Consequently, making sure that you include plenty of brain friendly foods in your diet, the kind of things that will help to make your brain tiptop condition such as oily fish like mackerel, salmon and anchovies (which are rich in Omega-3 essential oils) plus plenty of dark, leafy vegetables is a very good choice.

MICRO-MANAGING YOUR DIET

The idea behind micro-managing your diet is that even for people who would not necessarily agree that they are energy deficient all of the time, it may happen sometimes. For instance, there are certain times of the day when you really needs lots of energy, whilst other times, energy is far less essential. It therefore makes sense to feed your body with as much energy as it needs at the time when it most needs it, rather than doing so at times when energy is far less essential.

It is for this reason that many nutritional experts suggest that the most important meal of the day is breakfast, because a healthy, hearty breakfast sets you up for the day and provides you with the energy you need to get going. At the same time, most people who work a full-time job also need energy in the afternoon as well, and a reasonable lunch is also essential.

At the end of the day however, energy is far less important because after you have dealt with the rigors of the day, your body naturally starts to slow down as bedtime approaches. This is therefore the time of the day when the smallest amount of energy is needed. And yet, most people grab an apple as they charge out of the door in the morning, race through lunch before eating a big dinner when they get home.

In other words, in terms of providing the necessary

energy to keep you going, what you are doing is completely the wrong way round if this is what you do. A healthy balanced breakfast provides you with the energy you need to get over or through what is usually the hardest part of the day, whilst following this with a balances lunch should be sufficient to provide your body with energy you need to get through the afternoon as well.

It is however a fact that some people feel an almost overwhelming urge to have a nap in the afternoon, and unfortunately, if you are at the office or factory, this fact does not make this "I need a nap" feeling go away. Nowadays, there are some more enlightened companies who are beginning to recognize this fact. They have accepted that allowing employees to have a 15 to 20 minute nap is far better than having a drowsy employee who is incapable of achieving anything for an hour or two, but these organizations are not yet the majority, and probably never will be.

Hence, what you should do is eat a lunch that is designed to prevent you feeling sleepy afterwards. To do this, try to avoid carbohydrates at lunchtime. Focusing instead on a lunch that is predominantly protein-based. This works because proteins are broken down in your digestive system into amino acids, one of which is tyrosine which is known to keep you sharp and alert. Hence, instead of a carbohydrate packed lunch (which releases serotonin into your brain, a hormone that relaxes you9, aim to eat something that is protein rich such as a tuna and boiled gg salad or steamed fish and vegetables. Another idea that is very popular but not scientifically proven) is that some herbal supplements can help to overcome a temporary energy deficit, with many people swearing by garlic capsules or tablets, gingko biloba or ginseng.

The fact that all of these 100% natural substances seem to be capable of reviving energy levels without reverting to potentially harmful substances like processed sugar and are convenient to carry and take makes this another option that you might like to consider.

THE MENTAL SIDE IS IMPORTANT TOO

As I highlighted at the beginning of the book, your psychological state can play a very significant role in dictating how energetic you feel. If for example you are under constant stress, it is far harder to maintain a positive attitude and without a positive attitude, most people would find it very difficult to be energetic and enthusiastic. Hence, you need to decide whether there is a psychological reason why you don't feel as if you have any energy, starting with the obvious suspects such as stress and lack of sleep.

What's the root of the problem ?

Of you cannot sleep, it may be because you are stresses, but if you haven0t had any sleep for a couple of days, it becomes far more likely that you will feel stresses as your temper and general demeanor suffers. You therefore need to identify what is the root cause of your problem, because if you can do this, then it becomes relatively easy to deal with.

For example, it might seem almost too blindingly obvious but the reason why people sometimes cannot sleep is because the bedroom is not as dark as I should be. Even though this might sound like a relatively minor thing, it is truth, because if there is too much light, it interferes with your brains ability to handle melatonin secretion which is the hormone that is responsible for your body clock.

From this it follows that the darker your bedroom is, the more relaxed your sleep is likely to be which in turn guarantees that you will wake up in the morning completely revitalized and full of energy. This is one reason why some people wear eye shades in bed as it ensures that they get the full eight hours of uninterrupted sleep which most people need to remain energetic and enthusiast. As mentioned before, foods that are rich in carbohydrate release serotonin which help to relax and calm you down, so carbohydrate rich foods from an ideal pre-bedtime snack (in moderation) are a great way to end your day. Some people also find that a warm bath, perhaps with an infusion of aromatic oils helps to calm and relax them before bed too, so this is something else that you could try id a lack of sleep seems to be causing energy problems during the day.

DEALING WITH STRESS

Stress is a terribly debilitating condition, one that literally drains you of the very last drop of energy and vitality, as well as playing an active role in causing many potentially fatal conditions such as heart attacks and strokes. Hence, whilst fighting against stress to combat the lack of energy that you feel is important, it is probably not the most important reason for doing so. The basic idea behind most strategies for combating stress is that stress comes about because a situation or scenario prompts you to be physically unhappy or uncomfortable. It is often characterized as being the modern version of the "fight or flight" reaction to danger or a threat would have been understood by our caveman forbears. This in turn means that if you could teach yourself or somehow learn to react to external stimuli in a more positive way, then stress and the negative effects it has on you psychological (and ultimately physical) well-being would be minimized or banished forever.

In essence, therefore, dealing with stress is something that you have to learn, and there are several widely recognized ways of doing so.

The first strategy that you might consider using for dealing with stress is by using hypnotherapy, the medical version of hypnotism. Whilst there is still a good degree of mystery attached to why hypnotism works in the way it does, it is generally believed that when someone is in a hypnotic trance, the hypnotist or hypnotherapist who has induced the trance is able to communicate directly with the hypnotized subjects subconscious mind. The relevance of this is that by the time you reach adulthood, the way you react to specific situations is almost a subconscious reaction, something that you don't even think about. To understand this concept better, think of it this way. A newborn baby is a blank canvas as he or she has learned literally nothing about the world. Thus, if an axe wielding madman were to charge headlong at this newborn character, they would probably stare at this wild eyed onrushing figure with mild bemusement.

In contrast, you and I would prepare to fight or (more likely) run away because this is a conditioned reaction that we have learned over the years, and conditioned reactions come from the subconscious mind. Hence, because a hypnotherapist has the ability to communicate directly with your subconscious, they can analyze why you react in a stressed way to certain situations and conditions before changing your beliefs an reactions by communication directly with the root cause of them. Many people over the years have found that hypnosis or hypnotherapy is extremely effective for dealing with a wide range of subconscious reflex reactions such as minimizing the worst effects of stress because hypnotherapy has the ability to remove the trigger that prompts the reaction. Consequently, if you are a person who suffers stress which seems to be draining all of your energy, this is definitely an option to investigate. To do so, the easiest way of finding a locally qualified professional is to use google maps to run a search. An alternative that you might want to consider is to investigate the idea of self-hypnosis or using hypnosis products that you can buy on the net. Although you might be a little skeptical when first introduced the concept of self-hypnosis, there are lots of websites where there is plenty of information about it and more importantly, about how successful it can be.

For example, here are some instructions on how you can hypnotize yourself:

How to Perform Self Hypnosis

Self-hypnosis is a naturally occurring state of mind which can be defined as a heightened state of focused concentration. With it, you can change your thinking, kick bad habits, and take control of the person you are— along with relaxation and destressing from everyday life. It's similar to meditation and results in a better you.

Part 1 of 3: Preparing for Hypnosis

1

Get into comfortable clothing. It's pretty hard entering any kind of deep, relaxed state when all you can think about is the waistband of your jeans cutting off your circulation. So take this as an excuse to throw on some sweats. You want absolutely nothing distracting you.

- Make sure the temperature is good, too. Have a blanket or a sweater ready if you run on the chilly side. Sometimes feeling warm can be very comforting, too.

2

Go to a quiet room and sit in any comfortable chair, couch, or bed. Although some people prefer to lie down, you are more susceptible to sleep than when sitting up. Whether you sit or lie, ensure that you do not cross your legs or any part of your body. You may be in this position for a while and this could end up being uncomfortable.

3

Make sure you are not going to be disturbed for at least half an hour. No self-hypnosis is effective if it gets interrupted by a phone call, a pet, or a kid. Turn off your phone (and the alerts), lock the door, and sequester yourself. This is *you* time.

- The amount of time you want to dedicate to this is up to you. Most prefer to be in a trance (we try to avoid that phrase as it has certain...err...negative connotations) for about 15 or 20 minutes, but you have to allot time to get in and out of it, too.

4

Figure out your hypnosis goals. Are you doing it just to relax? For self-improvement? To train your brain? If you're doing it to achieve a greater end (weight loss, quitting smoking, etc.), prepare a list of affirmations. Self-hypnosis can be used just for relaxation, sure, but it can be for a number of life-enhancing things, too. Many use it to achieve their goals, change their thinking, or just as general positive reinforcement or motivation. Here are some examples of affirmations you could try:

- If you want to quit a bad habit, something to the point is the most effective. Think along the lines of, "I do not want to smoke. Cigarettes have no appeal to me."

- If you want to think more positively, aim for something like, "I am capable of whatever I set my mind to. I am in control and I am valuable."
- If you want to reach a specific goal, like weight loss, say it in the *present* tense: "I am eating healthy. I am losing weight. My clothes feel better and I feel better."
- These are statements you will be reciting to yourself when you're under. Again, it's up to you, but many find them life-affirming and effective.

Part 2 of 3: Entering Hypnosis

1

Close your eyes and work to rid your mind of any feelings of fear, stress, or anxiety. When you begin, you might find it difficult not to think. You may find that thoughts keep intruding. When this happens, don't try to force the thoughts out. Observe them impartially, and then let them slip away. See How to Meditate for more help with this step.

- Alternatively, some like to pick a point on the wall and focus on it. It could be the corner, it could be a smudge, it could be wherever you want it to be. Focus on the point, concentrating on your eyelids. Repeat to yourself that they're getting heavier and heavier and let them close when you cannot keep them open anymore.

2

Recognize the tension in your body. Beginning with your toes, imagine the tension slowly falling away from your body and vanishing. Imagine it freeing each body part one at a time starting with your toes and working its way up your body. Visualize each part of your body becoming lighter and lighter as the tension is removed.

- Relax your toes, then your feet. Continue with your calves, thighs, hips, stomach and so on, until you've relaxed each portion, including your face and head. Using imagery techniques of something you find comforting or soothing, such as water (feel the water rushing over your feet and ankles, cleansing them of tension) can be effective as well.

3

Take slow, deep breaths. When you exhale, see the tension and negativity leaving in a dark cloud. As you inhale, see the air returning as a bright force filled with life and energy.

- At this point, you can use visualization as you so choose. Think of a lemon and cut it in half in your mind. Imagine the juices oozing out and getting over your fingers. Place it in your mouth. What's your reaction? How does it feel, taste, and smell? Then, move onto more meaningful visions. Imagine your bills blowing away in the breeze. Imagine you running off those pounds. Get as detailed as possible. Always think of your five senses.

4

Appreciate the fact that you are now extremely relaxed. Imagine you are at the top of a flight of 10 stairs which at the fifth step start to submerge into water. Picture every detail of this scene from the top to the bottom. Tell yourself that you are going to descend the stairs, counting each step down, starting at 10. Picture each number in your mind. Imagine that each number you count is further down and one step closer to the bottom. After each number, you will feel yourself drifting further and further into deep relaxation.

- As you take each step, imagine the feel of the step under your feet. Once you are at the fifth step imagine and truly feel the refreshing coolness of the water and tell yourself that you are stepping into an oasis of purity and cleanliness. As you begin to descend the last five steps, start to feel the water getting higher and higher up your body. You should now start to feel somewhat numb and your heart will start to race a bit, but notice it and let any qualms about the situation just drift away into the water.

5

Feel a floating sensation. At this point at the bottom of the water you shouldn't really feel anything, just the sensation of floating freely. You may even feel like you're spinning. If you do not feel as stated above, try again, slower with a will to grasp what is happening. Once you have achieved this state you should proceed to address your problems and decide upon what it is you want from where you are.

- Now start to narrate what you are doing; speak in the present and future tense quietly to yourself, or as if you are reading it from a page.

- Start to picture three boxes under the water that you have to swim to get to. Once you have found the boxes, open them slowly, one at a time, and narrate to yourself what is happening when you open the box. For example, "As I open the box I feel a radiant light engulf me, I feel it becoming a part of me. This light is my new found confidence that I can never lose as it is now a part of me" and then proceed on to the next box.
- You should avoid using statements with a negative connotation, such as "I don't want to be tired and irritable." Instead, say, "I am becoming calm and relaxed." Examples of positive statements include: "I am strong and slender," "I am successful and positive," and, if you have pain, "My back is beginning to feel wonderful." (See warning on pain.)

6

Repeat your statement(s) to yourself as many times as you wish. Feel free to wander about the water, visualizing yourself emptying boxes, finding treasure (in the form of self-confidence, money, etc.), or simply letting all your tensions disappear.

Find areas where the water is cold, hot, or full of wildlife. Let your imagination go.

7

Get ready to exit your hypnotic state. With each step you take, feel the water becoming lower and lower until you have once again reached that fifth step. Once you are out of the water and are on the sixth step you may start to feel heavy or as if there is a weight on your chest. Merely wait on the step until this passes, constantly repeating your aforementioned statements.

- Once it passes, continue up the stairs, visualizing each step by its number, feeling the steps underneath you. Will yourself to carry on up the stairs.
    - For the record, this water visualization isn't 100% hard and true. If you come up with another scenario that you prefer, use it! It's

just as good, if not better, since it works for *you*.

8

Once you have ascended, give yourself a few moments before opening your eyes. You may want to visualize yourself opening a door to the outside world. Do this slowly and imagine the light that pours in through the doorway; this should make your eyes open naturally. If you need to, count down from ten, telling yourself that once you finish, your eyes will open.

- Take your time getting up. Then tell yourself, "Wide awake, wide awake," or something you're used to to wake up. This will put your mind back in the conscious state, bringing you back to reality.

Part 3 of 3: Enhancing Your Experience

1

Mean it. No self-hypnosis or mantra will manifest itself in real life if you don't actually mean it. In order for this to be effective, you have to believe in yourself and your actions. And why not? If you do mean it, it could work.

- If the first time doesn't seem effective, don't write it off automatically. Some things take time to get used to and to get good at. Come back to it in a few days and revisit the experiences. You may be surprised.
- Open your mind. You have to believe there is a possibility of this working in order for it to work. Any skepticism on your part will impede your progress.

2

Test yourself physically. If you need proof you're
in a trance, there are exercises you can do!
Anything that can be seen or felt in your body can
work. Try these ideas on for size:

- Entwine your fingers together. Keep them
  together throughout your trance, telling
  yourself that they are stuck together --
  almost as if they're covered in glue. Then,
  try to take them apart. If you find you
  can't...proof!
- Think of one arm getting heavier and
  heavier. You don't need to consciously pick
  one; your brain will do this for you. Imagine
  a book on top of it, holding it down. Then,
  try to lift it up. Can you?

3

Visualize situations. Whatever it is you're working toward -- be it confidence, weight loss, positive thinking, whatever -- visualize yourself in the situation acting as you'd like to react or being as you'd like to be. If you want to be thinner, imagine yourself sliding into your skinny jeans with ease, modeling in the mirror, smiling at your beautiful body. The endorphin rush alone will be worth it!

- Many use hypnosis to get over certain issues like shyness. You don't have to attack the shyness head on; something related will do. Simply imagining yourself going about the world with your head high, smiling, and making eye contact can be the first step toward a more extroverted you.

4

Use outside things to assist you. In other words, some people like music to help them enter hypnosis. There are a bunch of hypnosis tracks available online that are just for this purpose. If a certain scene -- water, the rainforest, etc. -- would help, you have it at your fingertips!

- Timers can be helpful, too. Some find that getting out of the trance is difficult and they lose track of time. If you don't want to accidentally spend hours hypnotized, you can use a timer. Just make sure it has a soothing tone to get you out of it.

5

Use it to better yourself. Find a goal of yours you'd like to achieve and concentrate on it during your relaxed state. Think of the person you'd like to be and be that person. Hypnosis is great for a deep, deep meditation, but it's better in that it can be used for a bigger, better purpose. Many people find that they emerge more positive and with a sense of purpose afterward. Take advantage of that possibility!

- There is no wrong way to go about this. Whether it's kicking a bad habit, having focus in your work life, or just changing your thinking, hypnosis can help. Getting rid of the stressors in your life is an integral part of being the person you want to become and this will help. And the more you do it, the better and more natural it'll feel.

Tips

- If you can't sleep, after you count down from ten (or go down your staircase), allow your mind to remain in this pleasantly relaxed state and keep your eyes closed while you are lying down and you will sleep much easier.
- Have an idea of how you will present your suggestions to yourself before you lie down and are relaxed, otherwise it may interrupt your hypnotic state.
- Another way to relax your muscles is to physically tense and hold for ten seconds before releasing; you should feel as well as imagine the tension leaving.
- Some find that imagining yourself in a peaceful natural setting will relax your mind sufficiently before counting down. For instance, you may imagine yourself wandering through a forest,

smelling the trees and hearing the wind. Alternatively, you could imagine yourself walking along the ocean shore and feel the grit of the sand beneath your feet, the cool water washing against your ankles and sounds of the surf.

- Don't force yourself or think about it and it will be much easier. Also this is a good way to get to sleep.

- Writing out your suggestions before induction can be very effective, as a visual list of what you choose to work on can sometimes be more easily remembered than even carefully assembled thoughts.

- For those of you who like to meditate but can't sit still long enough, just use this as a form of meditation but insert a period of time in between counting down from ten and counting back up to ten.

- If you are struggling, try visiting a hypnotherapist or buying a recording in order to experience hypnosis. When you have experienced it once or twice you will better know the state of mind you are aiming to achieve.

- It often helps to go to a professional, licensed hypnotherapist for a session first, to see what it feels like.

Warnings

- Be careful when rising if you've been lying down. Getting up too quickly could cause your blood pressure to plummet, and you could easily become dizzy or pass out. (This has nothing to do with hypnosis, it is orthostatic hypotension.)
- Hypnosis does not always work immediately; you may need to repeat it often (e.g. every day for a month or more) to see the benefits. You will need to "train" yourself with lots of practice.

Things you'll need

- ☐ A comfortable place to sit or lie down. Subdued lighting and the correct room temperature.

- ☐ A quiet environment where you will not be disturbed for at least half an hour.

Alternatively, try running a search for hypnosis products, because there are although 400,000 sites where you can buy hypnosis tapes, CD's, videos, books and everything you could think of that could be associated with hypnosis.

The basic idea of hypnosis as a way of dealing with stress is that through mastering your subconscious reactions, you learn how to relax instead of reacting in a stressed manner. A similar thing can be associated with another strategy that many people use to conquer their tendency to react in a stressed manner, which is to use yoga together with the associated practice of meditation and deep breathing to learn to overcome their susceptibility to stress.

Once again, if you are a person who suffers stress and you therefore find that your general levels of energy are not as good as they could be, this is another option which you can either learn from others in a controlled environment or start the ball rolling in the comfort of your own home via the medium of the net. Again it really doesn't matter where you live, there will be yoga class somewhere in the neighborhood and as before, you can find these quickly and easily by using google maps. As the google information includes the addresses, telephone number and of course the map. It enables you to contact them to establish whether they are in a position to help without stepping out of your front door. The other way of doing this is to start learning yoga from the net from any one of a number of sites that are focused on both the physical and the mental side of learning about ancient Eastern practice.

The basic idea of yoga is that by learning to control the way your mind reacts to situations and circumstances, you can achieve a far higher level of relaxation than you have previously managed. Consequently, as there is such a focus on mind control associated with yoga (primarily through meditation), it is an ideal pastime for anyone who suffers a lack of energy caused by reacting in a stressed manner to external stimuli.

The basic exercises attached to yoga are categorized by participants striking stationary poses that are designed to improve muscle flexibility and strength. These poses are known as Asanas and they range in difficulty from being relatively easy to very hard.

Hence it is important that if you would like to start investigating whether yoga is for you from home, you should use a site where the degree of difficulty is noted so that you do not attempt something that may cause physical damage or injury.

As far as the spiritual side of yoga is concerned, there are many different types of meditation associated with different forms of yoga, most of which come from different religions. There are also resources like meditation CD's as well as meditation supplies which can help you to meditate successfully.

The final thing that is intrinsically linked to yoga is having the ability to breathe deeply and slowly on demand because once you can do this. You have the capacity to take control of even the most stress inducing situation by forcing yourself to breathe properly. The importance of this can be demonstrated by the fact that most people in a stressful situation will breathe quickly and shallowly, which immediately limits the supply of oxygen to the brain and to the body. This in turn makes a situation that was already becoming difficult considerably more so. In this scenario, by starving your brain of oxygen, you have naturally limited your capacity to make well-reasoned, logical decisions, hence rapid breathing always exacerbates an already stressful situation.

Almost everyone who learns the art of deep breathing reports that as part of the learning process, they acquire the ability to be conscious of when stress is starting to happen and the fact that their breath is becoming quicker and more shallow at the same time. Once they acquire this level of consciousness, it becomes far easier to control their breathing, thereby bringing stress under control as well.

As there is with meditation, there are many different ways of learning deep breathing but using the Pavlov method is one that you should definitely consider because it is again focused on conditioning your subconscious mind which as established earlier is where stress comes from.

Learn Deep Breathing through Pavlov method

The Pavlov Method of Deep Breathing : This method of deep breathing is based on the technique used by Great Russian Scientist Ivan Pavlov (1849-1936) while introducing the concept of 'conditioned reflexes' .We will take the help of these 'conditioned reflexes' to make an unconscious habit of deep breathing.

First of all, let us see what are these 'Condition reflexes'

There are many actions (process) in our body which are not in our control. They happen on their own. Like beating of heart, digestion, circulation of blood etc. Breathing is also a process which is beyond our control. 'Conditioned reflexes' are the tools with the help of which we can control some of these seemingly uncontrolled process.

Let us understand these 'conditioned reflexes' in some more detail.

Pavlov did an interesting experiment on dogs. He noted that whenever he gave food to dogs, they started salivating(the secretion of salivary glands in mouth in the anticipation of food) and their digestion process started. He noted that whenever dogs saw that food is coming, the salivation started in their mouth.

Pavlov wanted to know whether this process of salivation and digestion in dogs can be influenced by any external factor (stimuli).

So he did a little experiment. He started ringing a bell while giving food to dogs. Whenever, he gave food to dogs, he rang a bell. He repeated this process regularly for some time. Slowly dogs become accustomed to this habit. Whenever they heard the sound of bell, they took it as the sign of food coming.

One day, at the time of food, Pavlov rang the bell. The dogs became attentive in anticipation of food. However, Pavlov didn't gave them food. He just rang the bell. However, he noted that dogs still started salivating and their digestion process started even in the absence of food.

Now salivation is a process which is not in our control. It happens on its own whenever we saw or eat food. However, in this experiment, the sound of bell started the salivation process in dogs. What actually had happened was that the brains of dogs began to associate the two incident of 'ringing a bell' and 'serving of food' together. Since they are occurring simultaneously, the brain of dogs took the mere sound of bell as the indication for food even when no food was served. This process in which the brain began to associate the ringing of bell with food is known as conditioning.

We will use this conditioning to make a habit of deep breathing.

Using 'Conditioned Reflexes' for Deep Breathing

There are many physical and mental activities which we perform almost daily. Like walking, eating, drinking, bathing, driving, cleaning our teeth, driving, reading newspapers & books, surfing the net, playing an indoor or outdoor game etc . The list is endless. The main thing is that we perform these activities almost daily. Right ?
We will use these activities as external stimuli to train our nervous system (mind) to automate the process of deep breathing.
Let us take 'Walking'. Every day we walk. We walk for different purposes in different places. We walk in a park in the morning, we walk to the market, we walk in our house, to the bus stand, to our boss's room, to attend a meeting or prayer, to meet someone somewhere and in many many other circumstances of life. We may use this walking activity to learn deep breathing.

Whenever we walk, it is for a purpose. We walk in the Garden early morning basically for the purpose of good health. We walk to the market for the purpose of buying something. We walk to bus stand or Railway Station for the purpose of reaching somewhere. We walk in our home for many purpose. We walk to our boss's room for some official purpose, we walk to meet someone, somewhere for a purpose. We walk into the bathroom for the purpose of bath. In short almost always whenever we walk it is for a small or big purpose. Agree ?

So what you have to do is to choose any purposeful walk. Just one. It may be the walk in the morning, or walk in the office, walk to the bus stop or any other purposeful walk. Now, whenever you walk for that particular purpose, breathe deeply. I mean whenever you walk for that purpose , give proper attention to your breathing and be aware of the inhalation and exhalation process. While walking for that specific purpose, try to breath as deeply as you can.

The important thing is that breathe deeply only (and always) when you walk for that particular purpose. For all other occasions of walking (and for other physical and mental activities) forget about this deep breathing and take breath in the way you normally do. However, whenever you walk for that particular purpose, breathe deeply.

Understand it with an example. Suppose you choose to breathe deeply while walking to the bus stop for the purpose of catching the bus. Now whenever, you walk to the bus stop, breathe deeply while walking. Give proper attention to your breathing while you walk and breath as deeply as you can. After catching the bus, restore the normal breathing and forget about this deep breathing. Repeat this process daily. Initially, it will be difficult. Often you'll forget about deep breathing. However, please remember that you are not required to breathe deeply throughout the day. Only when you walk to the Bus-Stop for catching the bus, you have to take deep breathing. It's not that difficult. Is it ? All of us can do it easily. It is true that initially you'll have to make conscious efforts for breathing deeply while walking to the bus stop, but soon your mind will be conditioned for this automatically.

Just as in Pavlov's experiments the dogs started salivating on hearing the bell, in the same way soon you will start breathing deeply automatically as you walk to the bus-stop.

Please don't think that I am comparing you with dogs (if some of you are thinking that way) I am just trying to tell that this Pavlov experiment can be very very useful for us in controlling the unconscious process of deep breathing.

The automatic arrival of Conditioned reflex

Do you know what you will be doing while you choose to take deep breath while walking for the purpose of catching a bus? You unconsciously train your mind to start associating the 'process of deep breathing' with 'walking to the bus stop'. Slowly the simultaneous process of 'walking to catch a bus and 'deep breathing' will become automatic. You'll see that even when you forget to breathe deeply while walking to bus stop, your mind reminds you automatically to breathe deeply. In other words a 'conditioned reflex, will be created in the form of that 'purposeful walk to the bus stop. Whenever you take a walk to catch a bus, you'll start breathing deeply on your own.

Now this is just one example involving a very small portion of your daily activities. Once you perfect this small deep breathing lesson, you can apply it in your other regular activities also. For example you can choose another purposeful walk. Let's say - choose the walk in the morning or 'an after meal walk' in the evening. Whenever you go for this walk, breathe deeply and slowly an association will be created between this walk and deep breathing. You can try other activities also. For example you can choose eating. Whenever you eat anything, breathe deeply. Give attention to your inhalation and exhalation process while eating. Slowly an association will be formed between the process of 'eating' and 'deep breathing' and you'll start breathing deeply as soon as you start eating anything. Apply this experiment of association on other activities of your daily routines. After a practice of two -three months, you will be able to create many association between deep breathing and your daily activities which in turn will add up to yours taking 3-4 hour of deep breathing daily. Taking such a good amount of pure oxygen than the amount you would take normally (i.e. without breathing deeply) will give you an unbelievable jest and energy. Not only your internal metabolism will improve but your overall physical and mental efficiency will improve greatly. This means less wear and tear of body, less exhaustion, less weakness and more vitality along with an enhanced capacity to work more.

Of all the yogic arts, deep breathing is the simplest and most efficient. It can be done anywhere, anytime with no restriction.
Having learnt about 'Deep Breathing' the first yogic aid in meditation, let us learn about the second powerful aid in meditation: Deep Relaxation

Deep Relaxation (Yog Nidra) :
Learn to relax yourself completely at will !
Most of us have forgotten the art of relaxation
Consider this :

Nomadic peoples all over Asia, journeying night and day, reach an oasis or camping place and at once throw themselves on the ground and lie there limp, apparently lifeless from head to foot. One hour of this rest refreshes them with as much new vitality and energy as a night's sleep for the average person. These wanderers are able to undertake surprisingly long journeys with very little rest. These people have not yet forgotten the art of relaxation, the ability to completely rest at will. This art has been practiced by yogis since ancient times. They began their experimentation on this state by watching animals in deep relaxation during sleep, and especially during hibernation.

Do you want to learn this art of deep relaxation ?

Let me tell you an ancient yogic method of deep relaxation (also known as Yog Nidra means the yogic sleep) It is strongly recommended for anybody who wants to learn meditation and is leading a very busy and demanding life to learn the art of deep relaxation. Since we all get exhausted (both physically and mentally) by the end of the day, it is very necessary for us to learn this art of deep relaxation. so that we an meditate with full vigor and enthusiasm.

Since we all get very tired and enervated in our daily routine, I am telling you a deep relaxation technique which is also a very powerful meditation. This technique serve the dual purpose of relaxation and meditation simultaneously. This is not only a very simple technique but also a very effective way to completely rest our body and mind.

Most of us spend our day in rush hour. The minute we wake up till the minute we go to bed, our body is subjected to immense physical and mental pressure. In such condition it is natural when we go to bed, we are completely exhausted and enervated. When people say they feel like crying with sheer fatigue, they mean just that. Physically, they have reached a point where the only release for their weariness is an emotional purge. Afterwards, of course, they will end up completely exhausted, for nothing eats up one's energy like letting the emotions have full play.

We keep losing energy every moment

Most of us are spendthrift of our energy resources. We
dissipate them twenty-four hours a day. Just watch
yourself and the people around you. Can you sit still,
quiet and at ease, for ten or even five minutes? Or do
you fidget, shift about, cross and re-cross your legs,
drum with your fingers on the arm of your chair, rub
your neck, bite your lips? In a room full of people, is
there even one who is without nervous habits? If so, he
is a happy exception. Nor mind you, does this apply to
"busy-busy" persons alone.
 it is perfectly possible to spend a quiet day with nothing
in the least urgent to do and still eat one's self up with
tension. In fact boredom itself is an enemy in this
respect. Think how many people with easy, routine jobs
complain of being "dead tired" by the end of the day.
And who of us hasn't said, at one time or another," I
haven't done a thing all day, but I'm beat."?

What is NOT relaxation ?

Before we go on to a discussion of the actual techniques
of Deep Relaxation, let us consider for a moment what
relaxation is not. In the first place, it is not play. Nor is it
a change of pace or of occupation. Play and change are

fine, of course. They do help, they are a step in the right direction. But they are not the real thing.

Thus the tired businessman out for a day of golf, the home gardener, the knitter, the Sunday painter are all people who indulge in pleasant hobbies in order to get away from other routines, but they are merely substituting one form of activities for another. The same holds true for the avid reader, the Hi-Fi enthusiast, the TV fan. Each finds a degree of respite in doing what he enjoys, but each remains occupied. The mind keeps ticking away, the muscles remain at work. Even listening to music with the eyes closed requires a certain expenditure of energy! Very definitely, recreation cannot be considered true, complete relaxation.

Understand what is true relaxation

The great art of relaxation is within the reach of all. It is better to understand it in detail. We use two kind of energy in our daily life - physical and mental. Overuse of physical energy results in exhaustion of physical body whereas use of mental energy results in an exhausted mind which specifically means exhaustion of our nervous system. In order to restore our vigor and replenish your energy , we need a relaxation exercise that helps us to relax us completely i.e. both mentally as well as physically.

A relaxation technique that that relaxes each and every muscle and every nerve of our body is Shava Asana ('Shuv 'Aa'Sun , Shuv sounds like 'love')

The Sanskrit meaning of Shavasan is Corpse Pose. It is not related to Death, only to hibernation, which has to do with the prolongation of life. It is an immense powerful technique for relaxing body and mind. This deep relaxation technique has far deeper effect than those of sleep. Moreover a very important meditation technique 'Death Meditation' is also based on it. This technique will relax you so deeply and so completely that it is impossible to sketch in words, the kind of vigor and energy you will received while doing it.

Instructions for Deep Relaxation

Before starting deep relaxation bear in mind that:

(1) Your aim is to quiet your nerves and rest your body by ridding yourself of all conscious tensions and contraction.

Deep relaxation is a must-do for all those who have the problems of :

(i) lack of vitality, fatigue, or poor concentration.

(ii) wearing oneself out by remaining constantly on the go with no moments of respite and never being able to gather enough energy for getting started on whatever they intend to do.

(2)To learn to relax completely takes time, and cannot be mastered in one easy lesson.

But you will certainly learn how if you are willing to try. Moreover, from the very beginning, even while you are still unable to let go completely, you will begin to feel the benefits of what you are doing. And this, in turn, will make for more success.

Soon your nervous system will become like a complicated network of highly charged electric wires with the current turned off: no hum, no sparks, no vibrations, while the batteries that are mainspring of energy recharge themselves.

Do you know that there are over four hundred muscles on each side of human body-no fewer than twenty in the forearm alone. Most of time we are not even conscious of using half of them. Moreover, we use them in groups and many of the small ones are beyond the range of our conscious feeling. Certainly we do not tense them consciously nor would we know how to let go of them

(3) Making a routine is very helpful in deep relaxation.

You should try, whenever possible, to do your relaxing exercises at approximately the same time each day. An early morning relaxation helps insure a good, serene day while a late evening period is a good preamble to a restful night's sleep. On the other hand, you might be one of those majority of people who need to replenish their energies at the end of their busy & tiring working day. In deciding what is best for you, your guide should always be your own ease and comfort. Any sense of "must", of pressure, should be avoided.

(4) Place of relaxation and cloths to wear during relaxation.

Unless you become so adept at relaxing that you can relax anywhere by shutting out the world around you at any time and any place, your period of relaxation should be taken away from other people, in a room where you are alone, with the door closed. You will need a quiet atmosphere so as not to be distracted by anybody. Since most of us are city dwellers it is difficult to avoid a certain amount of traffic noise, but do try to control what sounds you can, since conversation, the radio, the ticking of a clock can be most distracting. Keep disturbance at a minimum.

Your clothes should be comfortable, too. In fact, the less you have on the better : Make certain you are not annoyed by a tight belt, a stiff collar, a girdle, a brassiere. Anything that might make you unduly conscious of being physically confined should be avoided. On the other hand you must not feel cold. Be sure there are no drafts in the room since it is impossible to relax properly while chilly.

Now we'll start the real technique of deep relaxation:

The technique of Deep Relaxation

The best position for Deep Relaxation is Shavasana - the Corpse Pose. And the best place is the floor. Lie flat on your back, using a mat or folded blanket to protect yourself from the cold boards. If for some reason it is impossible for you to use the floor, then choose a hard bed, preferably one with a wooden board. A soft bed will never be completely satisfactory, for as it sags under your weight, certain muscles will invariably tense up.

Moreover, a soft bed might lull you to sleep, and sleep is not what you are after at the moment.

You will probably not feel entirely comfortable when you first try lying like this: The floor will feel too hard, you will find yourself tempted to shift positions. But this you must not do, for in order to relax muscle by muscle it is important to lie quite still.

Just remember that every body movement, every shift, however slight, means a tensing of one or another group of muscles To avoid this, make sure that you are lying comfortably, with your weight fairly evenly distributed.

Once settled take a few deep breaths from the diaphragm, then allow yourself to breathe normally again. The next step is to get acquainted with the muscles of your feet. Imagine that you have just swallowed a tracer substance, and that your muscles are channels through which you are watching it flow.

Now send an order along one of these channels. Breathe deeply and stretch a leg. Inhale deeply and stretch the leg hard, making all the muscles along the way contract- and feel what is happening . you will feel muscles, quite far away from the area with which you are experimenting, contract in sympathy. If you clench your fist, for example, you will feel contractions all the way up to your arm and into your shoulder. If you flex your toes, ripples of movement will tense the muscles of your thigh.

Now hold the breath as well as the stretch for a moment, while you trace your sensations in details. Memorize them: next time you give your arm an order you will be able to check whether or not it is being followed. And now let go. Release the breath and remove the stretch. As you exhale, let go all muscles of stretched leg loose. Repeat this simultaneous process (of deep breathing and stretching the muscles) limb by limb, until you have a nodding acquaintance with the various groups of muscles through your body.

Now start the stretching all over again, but this time in slow motion (i.e. make the process of inhalation and stretching slow) Build the stretch up, slowly, like a cat arching its back. In the meantime let that imaginary tracer substances show you, as clearly as possible, every muscle you have put into play. Observe and note your sensation for future reference. Hold the pose until you are thoroughly aware of what is happening. Then once more in slow motion, let go.

It is this letting-go process that is the actual mechanism of true relaxation. Think of yourself as a puppet without any strings to hold it up any longer. Could anything be more limp? That is the stage you are trying to reach, a relaxation so complete that you lose all feeling of alertness.

As I have already said you are not likely to achieve such state on your first attempt, or even on the second. Most people make better progress when instead of trying to relax the entire body at once, they concentrate on some part . Start for example, with an arm. Imagine that it is a length of old rope Let the shoulder fall inert, heavy, on the floor. Let the rest follow, all the way down the arm, until inertia has traveled through elbow, forearm, wrist and palm and the fingers feel like the limp ends of rope.

After doing this several times, start concentrating on your legs. Then on your neck and spine. After a while relaxation will become a habit and you will no longer need to think of specific areas, you will have learned to relax the entire body as a coordinated unit. When that time comes, you will be able to rest as you have never rested in your whole life. you will find a totally new sense of wellbeing; alertness and serenity.

A regular practice of this relaxation routine will make

you quite adept at doing this. Moreover, after you first feel thoroughly relaxed, you will find yourself capable of repeating the process on a deeper level - it is as though you had walked into a very quiet, deep forest, rested awhile, then walked on to where the trees are denser still and the silence deeper. In the end you will be on the very verge of drowsiness, of total inertia, your mind virtually at a standstill. When you reached that stage, you will be resting in every cell of your body.

The duration of deep relaxation

Well the time span of deep relaxation varies with its quality. The deeper the degree of relaxation, the more benefit you derive from it and the less time you need. Initially 15-30 minute is sufficient. Later on as you mastered the technique, you will able to draw enough energy and relaxation from a 10 minute period.

How to terminate the exercise ?

Well your own body will tell you when it is ready to get back into action. Remember, however, never to get up hastily or jerkily as doing so will negates the benefits of deep relaxation. The proper way to end a period of Deep Relaxation is to work your way down the muscles of the body one final time; but now by reversing the process.

Instead of relaxing, restore tone control to each muscle group. Contract or stretch it, then go on to another group until you have tested them all. Conclude with one final luxurious, cat-like stretch.

Why it is better than sleep ?

Please don't think that Sleep and deep relaxation are same in their benefits. Sleep whether, at night or during catnaps, is a fine way to rest the body. But it is the rare man or woman who relaxes thoroughly in sleep. Most of us toss and turn, and so continue tensing our muscle all night long.

Deep relaxation, on the other hand, since it is based on immobility, ensures total rest. It is a conscious, willed process, controlled by the mind which, in turn, relaxes thoroughly as the muscles begin to sag. In sleep we are likely to be fatigued by the dreams which plague our subconscious, for we all do dream, whether or not we remember our dreams. But resting while awake, after having emptied the mind of worrisome thoughts, means reaching a state of true mental repose. thus half hour of deepest relaxation can refresh an exhausted person as hours of fitful sleep never would.

If you can use any of these methods to successfully conquer your susceptibility to stress, you are immediately going to see a marked improvement in your energy levels as far less of your energy is wasted on futile stressful situations that you could not previously control. And of course, it should go without saying that as a part of your seven-day program to increase your energy levels, the sooner you start to control the stress you feel, the quicker you are going to start enjoying increased energy.

THE IMPORTANCE OF EXERCISE

One of the ironies of feeling that you have no energy is that fact that it discourages you from taking regular exercise. However, commencing a program of regular exercise is probably one of the best things you can do in terms of boosting your energy levels because the fact that exercise burns energy makes your body far more efficient at processing energy in the future.
Viewed from the opposite angle, if you do not do

exercise of some description, you are encouraging your body to be an inefficient machine for processing energy, which it will more than gladly do. But when you don't allow this to happen (i.e. when you exercise at least four times a week, your body gradually becomes fitter, healthier and a far more efficient energy processing plant, which of course means that if you exercise in this way on a regular basis, you will naturally feel more energetic, lively and vital.

What you really need is four sessions of cardiovascular or aerobic exercise every week as a minimum, something that works your heart, lungs , leg and arm muscles so that your whole body gets a workout.

Now, we are not talking about being an Olympic athlete here, nor am I suggesting that you go from doing no exercise whatsoever to trying to run a half marathon. Indeed, starting off with something as simple as a 15 minutes of brisk walking every day is a good idea because it is essential that you start off slowly and gradually build up, rather than going crazy from the beginning which is highly likely to cause injury.

Of course, the exercise program that you instigate will be dictated by your age and present physical condition, but you must nevertheless understand that if you want to feel more energetic and lively, taking up cardiovascular exercise is possibly the most important factor of them all. Exercise encourages your metabolism to speed up so that all of the energy from the food you consume is channeled in the right directions as an example of why this is so. At the same time, the fact that cardiovascular exercise involves movement will help every other process you have learned in this book to be more effective that it would otherwise be. For instance, even something as simple as walking prompts your digestive system to become more efficient because you are using the muscles of your upper legs, hips and buttocks, all of which are adjacent to the muscles that control your lower digestive system. Furthermore, it is an acknowledged fact that regular exercise improves oxygen flow to all of the organs of your body, including your brain, which helps to combat stress and tension. Indeed many people who take regular exercise report that doing so is one of the most effective ways of combating stress as it allows them to dissipate their aggression as they run, swim or cycle and it is natural that regular exercise will help you sleep better as well. As suggested, if you haven't exercised for some time, start off slowly with 15 minutes of brisk walking, if possible every day but failing this at least four times in your first week. Then add another 5 minutes in the second week, another 10 minutes in the third and so on until you can comfortably walk for an hour at a brisk pace.

At that point you might decide to accelerate the process

further by moving to jogging and then running, this is far more likely than it might appear right now because you will be feeling such noticeably elevated levels of energy that making a decision to step up a gear or two will seem like the most natural thing in the world.

Other options that are very good are cycling and swimming, with the latter being ideal for those who are a little older or perhaps not so strong because swimming uses every muscle in the body whilst there is no "impact" (with the attendant risk of injury) as there would be if you were pounding the streets jogging 5 miles every evening. In reality, as long as you are doing sufficient aerobic exercise, your energy levels will rapidly increase, especially if you combine this with anaerobic exercise by practicing yoga. You could for example practice yoga three times a week in combination with aerobic exercise four times a week so that you have a complete exercise program that is almost guaranteed to skyrocket your energy levels pretty much irrespective of whatever else you decide to do.

CONCLUSION

As you have read, there are lots of strategies that you can adopt that help combat a general feeling of listlessness or a specific feeling of tiredness and fatigue that comes over you at a particular time of the day. Nevertheless, because most people wo suffer from a lack of energy do so because of a combination of factors rather than any single thing that drains the energy out of them, I would suggest that you adopt the same approach to reversing the situation.

For example, if you start your organic fruit and vegetable fast tomorrow whilst combining it with the supplements that will help to clean out your system, it would also make sense to start looking into the viability of hypnotherapy or yoga and take tour first 15 minute walk as soon as you have finished reading there final few paragraphs.

And as highlighted, do not underestimate the power of exercise to re-energize your body and your mind. Walking or jogging when combined with yoga and even something as simple as stretching makes sure that your brain is getting the oxygen it needs to manage your body efficiently. But you are not going to get anywhere if you don't take action, and whilst I appreciate that taking action is possibly one of the last things you might want to do if you have no energy, you also know that without action, nothing is ever going to change.

You now have the tools you need to do the job. It is up to you to use them.

In combination with cleaning your body out at the same time, even the gentlest exercise makes it far easier for energy to be channeled in the most beneficial directions, so you will naturally feel re-energized remarkably quickly.

www.ingramcontent.com/pod-product-compliance
Lightning Source LLC
Chambersburg PA
CBHW071356280526
45787CB00001B/353

* 9 781517 507190 *